Praise for *Ego State Therapy*

An interesting and, in many ways, invigorating new look at Ego State
Therapy has been presented by Dr. Gordon Emmerson of Australia in his new
book. Dr. Emmerson takes the technique away from the usual neurosis
therapies and/or personality dysfunctions and strides into the realm of
developing innovative techniques with which to approach therapeutic
dilemmas, experienced by the patient/client as ambivalence, feeling 'stuck' in
old patterns of behavior and interactions, processing intrusive traumatic
experiences, and dealing with unwanted parts and aspects of the self.
– **Marlene E Hunter, MD, FCFP(C)**, Past President, ASCH, ISSD, CSCH(BC),
Director, LabyrinthVictoria Centre for Dissociation

Gordon Emmerson brings to contemporary Ego State Therapy a voice that is
creative, unique, and helpful. *Ego State Therapy* will undoubtedly serve as a
handbook for many who want to learn more of the 'hands on' aspects of this
form of treatment. He is to be commended especially for his applications of
Ego State Therapy to the difficulties of the 'walking neurotic'.
– **Claire Frederick, MD**, Editor, *American Journal of Clinical Hypnosis*, co-author
of *Healing the Divided Self: Clinical and Ericksonian Hypnotherapy for post-
Traumatic and Dissociative Conditions* and *Inner Strengths: Contemporary
Psychotherapy and Hypnosis for Ego-Strengthening*

Mind, matter and life are the three distinct factors that instil Man with
inconceivable possibilities, of which Ego forms a crucial part. Ego determines
whether he becomes his own creator or destroyer. In him are found both evil
and virtue, both criminal tendencies and saintly characteristics. He may
either be a blessing or a curse to himself and others. Thus the good old
saying, "some are wise and some are otherwise." *Ego State Therapy* by
Gordon Emmerson incorporates hypnotherapy and presents innovative
techniques of working with Ego States. The theories of Ego State and the
practical methods illustrated in this book will enable the reader to master the
therapy with ease and thus to harness his own resources. This book will be a
very valuable addition to the subject of Ego State Therapy.
– **Professor V. M. Mathew MBBS, DTM&H, DPM, MRCPsych, M.Phil**

This book will be a very useful addition to any therapist's library and particularly beneficial to those new to the profession, in that it will give them an even greater grasp of the technique known to many as "Parts Therapy". Although the book is, in essence, based on the Watkins' Ego State Therapy, the author has built on the technique and used innovative ways of expanding its use. Some of the case studies in the book are fascinating and are used to enable the reader to more easily understand how the technique works and the uses it can be put to. I must confess that I had never thought of using the therapy in some of the ways that the author does and can see that its use could be expanded in any number of different directions, thus enabling the therapist to do brief therapy with many clients who might have been considered too difficult to treat quickly.

Gordon Emmerson has drawn on some of the different therapies which use these techniques, including Transactional Analysis. Gestalt Therapy and Voice Dialogue Therapy and he illustrates how Ego State Therapy can be incorporated into and used alongside almost any discipline to very good effect.

I found this book very enjoyable and easy to understand and I felt as if I'd added considerably to my tool-box after reading it.

– **Pat Doohan**, FIDELITY _ The Journal for the National Council of Psychotherapists

Ego State Therapy is a rapid psychotherapeutic method which uses the recognized advantages of hypnosis to produce the lasting positive outcomes characteristic of psychoanalysis with intervention times rivaling cognitive-behavior therapy. Representing the new generation of Ego State Therapists, Dr. Emmerson casts the masterful development of the approach over the years by John G. Watkins and his associates into the first true textbook on Ego State Therapy that clearly, accurately and succinctly shows clinicians and advanced clinical psychology students how to use Ego State Therapy with their patients. Much more than a "how to do" approach, *Ego State Therapy* keeps the series of well developed and time proven specific interventions accurately grounded in the underlying theory. It will become a classic as an essential text for those psychologists and psychiatrists who recognize the importance of Ego State Therapy to the needs of their clients.

– **Professor Arreed Franz Barabasz, EdD, PhD, ABPP,** Washington State University, USA, Editor, International Journal of Clinical and Experimental Hypnosis, President, American Psychological Association Div. 30 Society for Psychological Hypnosis

We have all experienced good teachers in our time – someone who engages us, holds our attention and shares knowledge with us, filling us with enthusiasm for the subject. Gordon Emmerson is such a teacher. His practical approach of providing the theory of a technique, demonstrating the technique and then monitoring his students as they practice the technique is unsurpassed.

Gordon has successfully transposed his teaching expertise into this book that has been described as "a classic as an essential text". It is a book that meets the needs of all readers, regardless of their level of expertise in Ego State Therapy.

The author discusses the goals and benefits of Ego State Therapy and the nature, development and permanence of ego states. He includes the steps to be taken in numbered point form, offering a full explanation of each step and "demonstrates" with client/therapist dialogue. The only thing missing is for the author to be there when the student practices. At the end of the book, we are taken through 3 sessions; each step is fully explained and there is no holding back of information.

I have fulsome praise for this most welcome text that gives valuable insight into Ego State Therapy and a practical approach to using the techniques in one's practice.

– **Lyn Macintosh CMAHA ASCH**, *Hypnopatter, Official Newsletter of the Australian Hypnotherapists' Association*

A wonderful encapsulation of an approach to therapy that embraces the multi-level communication within our psychotherapeutic system. Students of Erickson and Gilligan will find further clarification of familiar processes and principles of healing through self-relating. Gordon Emmerson is another welcome voice in the movement of therapy that works to embrace and respect the forces of the unconscious/ego relationship, enhancing understanding, expression and tutilage of "parts" rather than removing or dismissing problem states as irrational or "unresourceful". Many scholared and experienced therapists believe that there are many psychotherapies but only very few core psychotherapeutic processes. If so, Emmerson has done much to elucidate the practice and application of one of these core processes that obeys the natural laws of psychotherapeutic recovery and growth and is drawn from experience, skilled technique and wide knowledge.

–**Pamela Gawler-Wright**, *Beeleaf Training, www.beeleaf.com*

Ego State Therapy is based on the premise that our personality is not a homogenous whole, but is formed of separate parts. This idea in itself is ancient - you can find it inferred in writers from Aristotle to Shakespeare. More recently it is echoed in the Parts Therapy approach which has its roots in the work of Fritz Perls and was further developed by Gil Boyne, Charles Tebbetts and Roy Hunter. Systemic therapists talk of our 'Inner Others', and Transactional Analysis has explored the term Ego States in a somewhat different way. The form of therapy that Emmerson describes derives from the work of John and Helen Watkins and is an eclectic mix with hypnosis being a strong ingredient.

A reader of this book would have a very clear idea of the theoretical underpinnings of this approach as well as a wide range of techniques available to them by the time they had finished with it. With my NLP background I am familiar with working with Parts (or Ego States) with techniques such as Visual Squash and the Core Transformation process, but this book gave me new ideas about how to extend the range of my interventions.

The detail provided is in-depth without ever being turgid, and would allow most practitioners to begin using this approach with confidence.

Instinctively I am against therapies that take one aspect of our humanity and claim it as the single route to cure. Emmerson avoids this, for all his obvious passion and commitment to Ego State Therapy, offering a range of possibilities for working with a range of issues that are commonly brought to the consulting room.

An intelligent, well-researched and well-written book. Put it on your wish list, but don't leave it there for long.

–**Trevor Silvester,** Hypnotherapy Journal

Ego State Therapy

Gordon Emmerson, PhD

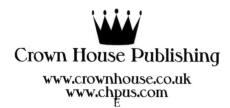

Crown House Publishing
www.crownhouse.co.uk
www.chpus.com

First published by

Crown House Publishing Ltd
Crown Buildings, Bancyfelin, Carmarthen, Wales, SA33 5ND, UK
www.crownhouse.co.uk

and

Crown House Publishing Ltd

6 Trowbridge Drive, Suite 5, Bethel, CT 06801-2858, USA
www.chpus.com

British Library Cataloguing-in-Publication Data
A catalogue entry for this book is available
from the British Library.

International Standard Book Number
978-1845900793

Library of Congress Control Number
2007932738

Printed and bound in the UK by
Anthony Rowe, Eastbourne

Dedication

I would like to thank Dr John Watkins and Helen Watkins (2002) for their hospitality, reading and wisdom during my sabbatical stay in Missoula while working on this manuscript; my two young sons Daniel and Dylan for their unceasing love and understanding; and two dear and loving friends Dan Ramsey and Delwyn Goodrick for their reading and encouragement. I would also like to thank Lyn Macintosh for her determination that this text be read.

Table of Contents

What lies in the dark unconscious expanse of our psyche?
What causes the words we hear in our mind?
What internal dynamic produces depression, panic attacks,
and addiction?
How can learning what is inside bring back the love and wonder
of childhood?

Foreword

It has been more than a century since Freud and his associates discovered unconscious mental processes. Other psychological pioneers, such as Janet, Binet and Prince, also made monumental contributions in this area, and a major psychological tradition called "Psychoanalysis" emerged. This approach stemmed from philosophical rationalism and was based on observations made of patients seeking help for mental conflicts, and on self observations through introspection.

Other seekers for human understanding, impressed by the contributions of the physical sciences, sought freedom from "subjectivism" by focusing on the "objective results" of mental processes, e.g., "behavior". Behavior was tangible and more easily lent itself to laboratory experimentation.

From these pioneers (which included James, Dewey, Thorndike, Watson and others) the second major psychological system, "objective empiricism" developed. Psychology re-defined itself as "the science of behavior".

This tradition dominated the psychology of the 20th Century. From it, brief, active systems of psychological treatment emerged, such as behavioral and cognitive therapy.

Each tradition had its own limitations. Psychoanalysts, relying primarily on free association, dream interpretation, and the analysis of transference reactions as their research "tools" developed a system of therapy, which, though often effective, required the expenditure of many hours of treatment.

Although psychoanalysis has continued, and has developed more sophisticated theories, (object relations, self theory, Lacanian psychology, etc.) there has been almost no change in the basic "tools" of its therapeutic technique. Accordingly, psychoanalysis has languished as a "practical" treatment modality.

The empirical-behavioral tradition, while showing immediate therapeutic results, has done so by ignoring conditions and behaviors which are mediated through sub-liminal, "unconscious" processes, thus severely limited the scope of its operational area. Also controversial, is the long-term permanence of symptomatic improvements achieved through cognitive-behavioral therapies.

Abandoned by psychoanalysts, and initially ignored by academicians (because of the ill-repute of stage demonstrations) clinical and experimental hypnosis has continued to occupy the focus of an active group of investigators and practitioners. Small in number, but sparked by such well-respected academicians as the Hilgards at Stanford University, and innovative therapists, like Milton Erickson and many others, this third tradition has continued and flourished. Their findings are publicized through several hypnosis journals and within national and international hypnosis societies.

In the past 30 years a small group of such hypnotherapists, seeking to develop a more rapid treatment methodology, which would combine the speed and efficacy of the cognitive-behavioral approach, plus the depth of the psychoanalytic tradition, have been developing a therapeutic system known as "Ego State Therapy".

Based on the psychoanalytic theories of Paul Federn, John and Helen Watkins and their associates (including Frederick, Phillips, Hartman, McNeal, Morton and others) have published many papers and several books detailing Ego State Therapy techniques. Other investigators, (such as Kluft, Torem, Fraser and Hunter) have further advanced the use of Ego State Therapy in the treatment of dissociation.

Moreover, the "First World Congress of Ego State Therapy" was held March 20–23, 2003, in Bad Orb, Germany, sponsored by German and European hypnosis societies.

Ego State Therapy promises rapid, long-lasting results in much shorter time than psychoanalysis, and several empirical, efficacy studies have already been published demonstrating its validity

(Watkins & Watkins, 1997, pp. 162–194; Emmerson, 1999; Emmerson & Farmer, 1996).

This present work, *Ego State Therapy*, by Gordon Emmerson is a major building block in the emerging body of literature which marks this developing approach. It is comprehensive in covering the field, and will be a basic reference on Ego State Therapy for years to come.

Newcomers to this approach sometimes have difficulty conceptualizing just what is meant by "an ego state". A strength of this work is the way Emmerson, using metaphors and other explanatory methods, clarifies just what an "ego state" is, and how it functions in the psychic economy of the entire person.

He clearly delineates states that represent more conscious moods, which he terms "surface" ones, and states that are normally below the threshold of awareness, for which he uses the term "underlying". These latter ones generally require hypnotic activation to make them accessible for therapeutic interventions.

While he does not severely criticize other systems of treatment he points out that the "cognitive therapies" must of necessity deal with "surface states", and he opts for more depth in therapy noting that, "to paste a coping skill on the surface of an injured personality is to further remove that person emotionally from 'Self'".

Emmerson presents the therapist/client verbalizations in many different cases, which help the reader to understand just how he, and his colleagues, practice Ego State Therapy.

In these, he himself often employs the Socratic-questionings commonly used by cognitive therapists. However, he demonstrates how much deeper insights can be achieved when these are administered to a "hypnotized" client, and he advocates the learning of hypnotic skills by more therapists.

The message here is that Ego State Therapy is not simply a specific, coherent treatment approach, but that its techniques can be adopted and added to the armamentarium skills of the cognitive therapist, the psychoanalytic therapist and other practitioners.

His text differs from that of the Watkins and Watkins (1997)[1] in that his broad experience has been apparently drawn from working with non-hospitalized private clients. His cases are more like those treated by Helen Watkins than the severe neuroses and dissociations which John Watkins encountered in military and Veterans Administration Hospitals. Thus, his cases and treatment techniques complement those found in the Watkins' text. The goals of insight, integration, and personality reorganization, however, are similar in both volumes.

Therapists and counselors will find this work an excellent and well-written textbook for the learning of Ego State Therapy – especially when combined with study in clinical hypnosis.

John G. Watkins, PhD
Professor Emeritus
University of Montana

---

[1] Watkins, J. & Watkins, H., 1997, *Ego States: Theory and Therapy*, Norton, New York.

Introduction

Turning the Lights On: Ego State Therapy

What is the ego? It is our awareness of the "me" inside. It is the "me" that is sometimes focused and working, sometimes playful and laughing, sometimes in pain, and sometimes illogical in feeling and reaction. We each experience our ego from our own special states, states that have been formed through our experiences.

Think about how you feel, right now, and point a finger to yourself. You are thinking about and pointing to your ego, your selfness, your "me state". You have more than a single "me state" or "ego state". You are made up of an ego family of states. At times you may feel like a different person in attitude, logic, and emotion. You are actually a single person who is made up of a number of different states; each has its own feeling of power, weakness, emotion, logic, or other personal traits. On another day or at another time, when you point to yourself, you will probably be pointing to a different ego state. The other state may be angry, logical, lighthearted, or fearful. It may be talkative or pensive. When we say, "Part of me wants to", we are talking about an ego state. When we say, "I feel at peace with myself on this issue", we are talking about our ego states agreeing, not having an internal struggle. Our various states help to make our lives rich, productive, and enjoyable.

Because we have many states from which we can choose at a given time, it is possible to learn to change from a state that feels out of control to a state that has a feeling of competence. Because we have states that carry pain, it is possible to find and help the specific states that need resolution. Working with ego states can foster an improved psychological and physical experience of life. Understanding these ego states, learning to recognize them, and to use them in therapy is the purpose of this book. Learning to work directly with the state that needs help provides therapists the shortest distance between the two points, the goal and the solution.

Goals of Ego State Therapy

The goals of the therapy are:

1. To locate ego states harboring pain, trauma, anger, or frustration and facilitate expression, release, comfort, and empowerment;
2. To facilitate functional communication among ego states (the statement "I hate myself when I am like that" indicates two states lacking in proper communication); and
3. To help clients learn their ego states so that the states may be better used to the clients' benefit (e.g., allowing the client to, at one time, be open to enjoy emotional experiences and, at another time, be assertive when challenged).

Benefits

Learning about ego states and how to use them is beneficial in two ways; it increases an understanding of personality, and provides an avenue for affecting rapid and lasting change.

Ego state personality theory allows the therapist and the client to have a clearer view of how the personality is composed, and where most psychological problems originate. It demystifies the "vast unknown subconscious", revealing it to be accessible ego states. It illuminates the development of our ego state structure and the ability that ego states have to be malleable, to become empowered, and to release fear.

Where do psychological problems come from? Why do clients react the way they do? Both clients and therapists often guess at these answers. Ego State Therapy provides a process that can connect the problematic symptom to the causal stimulus, without the therapist or client having to guess or interpret. It facilitates empowerment, just where it is needed, so unwanted symptoms no longer manifest from unresolved states. The understanding of their ego states that clients gain allows a richer experience of living, with an ability to be assertive, fragile, angry, logical, and caring at preferred times. Internal turmoil, where two parts of the person cannot agree, can be changed to a cooperative and respectful acceptance of the various ego states and their roles. It is often the case that physical health improves following the resolution of trauma and the improved internal communication between states that Ego State Therapy produces. Improved psychological and physical health, and an improved self-understanding and richness of experience are benefits of ego state theory and therapy.

Chapter 1 of this book defines ego states and ego state theory. It explains ego states and how the theory relates to other therapeutic orientations. A short history of Ego State Therapy is provided. Various ways to access ego states, both hypnotically and non-hypnotically, are presented in Chapter 2. Methods for using Ego State Therapy are covered in Chapter 3, and some specific applications of the therapy are presented in Chapter 4. Typical Ego State Therapy sessions are outlined in Chapter 5, and theoretical implications of ego state theory are discussed in Chapter 6.

Chapter 1

What are Ego States and How Did We Learn About Them?

Ego state therapy is based on the premise that personality is composed of separate parts, rather than being a homogenous whole. These parts (which everyone has) are called ego states. The state that is conscious and overt at any time is referred to as the executive state. Some non-executive ego states will be consciously aware of what is happening, while others may be unconscious and unaware. If a person is feeling and expressing anger, the executive state is a state that has as one if its roles, anger. The person may make statements such as, "I am really upset with you", or "You are no friend of mine". The angry person will own the feeling, saying "I" and will have the strong feeling of truth in what is said. The feeling is, "This is me, and this is what I feel". What is actually happening is feelings are being expressed by one ego state of the person. Other ego states (or parts) of the person may not have the same feeling. An hour later, when another ego state is executive the person may think and feel in a very different way, and statements may be made such as, "I don't know why I said those things. Your friendship is really important to me". At this time the feeling of "me" rests in a different ego state. A different ego state is executive.

The following examples will better demonstrate ego states.

I want to marry her: I don't want to marry her

Matthew is in a new relationship with Emma. He sees Emma playing with a child. He feels and believes, "This is the woman for me. I love her and want to spend the rest of my life with her." Later in the same day she criticizes him about his job as a plumber. He feels defensive and feels and thinks, "What did I ever see in this woman. How can I get out of this relationship?" These responses may sound extreme, but they are not unusual for many people, and it is

1

not unusual for a person to bounce among several ego states in the process of making a major decision (one state may be in favor, one may be against, and another indifferent). In one moment on one day Matthew may "know" he wants Emma as his partner, and in another moment he may "know" he does not. In this example Matthew has an ego state that loves and dreams of a family. It is a soft, caring part of him, and when he sees the woman he cares about playing with a child his "Loving/Caring" ego state becomes executive. While in this state, Matthew is capable of feeling very positive and interested in Emma. These are honest feelings. It is Matthew who is feeling them. It is Matthew's "Loving/Caring" part. Later when Emma criticized his job, another part of Matthew is energized to become executive (comes out). Matthew's "Defensive, don't pick on me" ego state becomes executive. This is not a loving, caring part of Matthew, and probably cannot even feel love. Its role is to protect, by creating a shell and withdrawing from the attacker. While in this state, Matthew cannot imagine a life with Emma. This, too, is a part of Matthew, just as valid and needed as the other. If Emma and Matthew continue with their relationship these two ego states will begin to differ less in the way Emma is viewed, but when he switches between them each will always reflect its role. His "Defensive" state will probably gain assurance over time that Emma will not hurt him, and either he will not switch to that state as much, or when he does his "Defensive" state will be less reactionary in its attempt to protect him.

Life is good: I want to hide

Lisa is having a good morning. She has just driven her new car to her adult education class. She has been admiring the new car and she feels good about having it. It makes her feel good to drive it. She is in an "I'm good" ego state. Lisa has not taken care to watch the time and when she enters her class she is 10 minutes late. The teacher stops talking to the group and states, "In the future I would really like it if everyone was here at the beginning of class." Lisa switches to a "Withdrawn" ego state, feels upset on the inside, and wants to shrink into a corner and hide. She feels exposed and in need of protection. She has negative feelings about herself, and about her ability to be a positive part of the group. Another person, or Lisa at another time, may respond in a very different way. We all have ego states particular to our own history. The ego state that becomes executive at a given time will depend on the activating events, and both on our recent history (how we have been feeling) and our complete history (what ego states we have developed and their relation to our other states). Lisa's switching states is a normal part of how we respond. We all switch states in relation to our life circumstances.

1.1   Ego States

An ego state is one of a group of similar states, each distinguished by a particular role, mood and mental function, which when conscious assumes first person identity. Ego states are a normal part of a healthy psyche, and should not be confused with alters (multiple personalities in dissociative identity disorder, see section 1.1.2, h). Ego states start as defense coping mechanisms, and when repeated develop into compartmentalized sections of the personality that become executive (conscious and overt) when activated. Ego states may also be traumatized during a single incident of trauma. For example, an ego state may be traumatized with an auto accident, a rape, a robbery, or even during the first day of kindergarten. Our unconscious contains our ego states that are not executive, and some ego states have not been executive for many years. They maintain their own memory and communicate with other ego states to a greater or lesser degree.

Suppose a parent verbally punishes a four-year-old child. The child may find that withdrawing, becoming quiet and saying nothing is a way to cope with the situation. The "Withdrawn" state becomes an ego state after the withdrawing behavior continues to work for the child on different occasions. Throughout life, when the person feels "in trouble with an authority figure" the withdrawn ego state may return, with the same feelings experienced by that four-year-old child. The adult may enter the same state when an authority figure rebukes or complains. Therapeutically, it is important to speak directly with the troubled ego state so a change can be made.

Hypnosis, with ego state techniques, allows this "Withdrawn" ego state to be accessed and spoken with. When asked how old it feels,

3

it responds with, "four". When asked, "What images do you have of being four?" the client will often regain the memory of that first incident of withdrawal (for more detail in accessing troubled states see section 2.2.5, The Resistance Bridge Technique). Work that assists that four-year-old state to feel resolved and empowered is usually permanent and allows the client to stop withdrawing when coming into contact with authority figures.

1.1.1   The Nature of Ego States

- An ego state cannot be eliminated, but it can be changed (see section 1.1.2, d).
- An ego state is normally able to express how old it feels. Usually it reports being younger than the client, although occasionally a state will say it feels older.
- Ego states may choose to hide or become inactive, and they can change. Sometimes when they change they prefer to have a new name ('Frightened' may become 'Helpful').
- Ego states, when asked, report they are a part of the person.
- Ego states have identity. When a state is executive (conscious) it speaks in the first person and speaks of other states as 'other'.
- Ego states have feelings, and do not like derogatory comments made about them, directly or to other states. They may refuse to talk or co-operate.
- We all have ego states, although the dissociation between them varies among individuals.

1.1.2   Development and Permanence of Ego States

We all have ego states and no two people have the same ego states in the same way. Our ego state map is the map of our personality. This section will address the following questions:

a.   How many ego states do we have?
b.   Where do ego states come from?
c.   What are surface states and underlying states?
d.   How long do ego states last?
e.   Can you get rid of an ego state?

f. Is there an age when we no longer develop new ego states?
g. What is ego state communication?
h. How do ego states differ from Multiple Personalities?

HOW MANY EGO STATES DO WE HAVE?

The average person has approximately 5 to 15 ego states that are used throughout the normal week. These states are close to the surface of the personality and usually communicate well with each other. When we switch from one to another we generally remember what happened and what we were doing in the previous state, although this memory is not complete. When we walk from watching television into the kitchen and open the refrigerator door we often switch from a relaxing/spectator ego state to a more functional/doer ego state. We are able to remember where we came from (the other room) and what we were doing (watching TV), but occasionally we may not remember why we came into the kitchen. When we sit for an exam in a nervous ego state we may not remember well the things we learned in a relaxed ego state, but if we are able to switch into the state we studied in, our recall will be much better.

Other than the few ego states we normally use, we have many more that we have used in the past, or that we rarely use. When walking along a street, if we notice a smell we have not smelled since childhood we may be flooded by childhood memories. A childhood ego state that used to experience that smell has been jogged into the executive, being energized by the "smell reminder". It would not be possible for a person to learn exactly how many ego states they have since some rarely come to the executive, but later in this book ego state mapping will be described. This is a process of naming and mapping the roles and communication lines of many of our ego states.

WHERE DO EGO STATES COME FROM?

A new ego state is created when a person is confronted with a frustration or trauma, and has no ego state that can respond. Most ego states start in childhood, and as the repertoire of states increases fewer are formed in adolescence, and fewer still in adulthood.

Lisa (from the introductory section) had an ego state called "Withdrawal". When Lisa was small she had a parent who would become very angry and yell at her. She found that by becoming quiet and looking small, the yelling would subside. This became a coping skill she used and continued to use. Since this withdrawal worked for her it became a part of her personality. Her 'Withdrawal' state learned to be cued to become executive when she felt "criticized by an authority figure". Later throughout her life her "Withdrawal" state would become executive during such criticism. This is what Freud called a situational neurosis. It is an inappropriate response to a life situation caused by an early trauma. The processing of early traumas in order to help free the person of related neuroses is explained in section 3.1.2.

Another example of ego states originating from usable coping skills is that of a child, Hank, who feels he is not getting enough attention from others. He tells a joke and finds this brings him the attention he needs. He tells other jokes, and says funny things, and gains more positive attention. A "Comic" ego state develops. Later in life when he feels a lack of attention he goes to his comedian ego state. This could be quite a positive ego state for him. Many of our states are positive and useful. We have states that allow us to feel love, to truly enjoy a sport, or a particular food. Smokers will have ego states that enjoy smoking and ego states that do not want to smoke. This is another example of two ego states wanting different things.

An ego state may change during a single trauma, such as a rape, or a bad accident, or a war trauma. If the trauma is repeated that ego state will often return, and it will probably return at other times, if related 'reminder' events occur. Sexual relationships may at times bring to the executive an ego state that experienced a sexual assault. The noise of a gun firing may bring to the executive an ego state that experienced a war trauma. Ego State Therapy allows the traumatized ego states to be brought to the executive and empowered so they may no longer have to negatively interfere with the person's life.

Ego state formation may be described using a metaphor. Imagine the young brain as smooth, fertile, loose soil on a gentle slope. It has no channels for water to run. A number of small rains combined, or fewer major rainstorm, will make channels that become permanent in this soil. The channeled hillside will naturally direct any water that falls near a channel into it. As the small child repeatedly uses a working coping mechanism a neural pathway is established in the brain and events that are reminders of that coping mechanism will be channeled down that pathway to the associated ego state. A trauma can be seen as the major rainstorm that can alter a channel in a single incident. Reminders of that trauma will bring to consciousness (the executive) the associated ego state.

WHAT ARE SURFACE STATES AND UNDERLYING STATES?
A distinction can be made between two types of ego states, surface states and underlying states. Surface states are those states that are most often executive in normal functioning. They have good communication between each other. This means that a surface state (e.g., one that is cognitive and deliberative) will remember what happened when a different surface state (e.g., one that is more emotional) was executive. There is relatively good memory between them. Daily routine is experienced by surface states.

Underlying states vary greatly in their relative closeness to the surface. Some very rarely become executive. Some have almost no communication with surface states. These states become executive only occasionally outside therapy. The person who sees a wall paper like that of a childhood room may experience an underlying ego state, bringing with it childhood feelings and memories. Some of these memories may have previously been unknown to the surface states. Clinically, underlying states are difficult to access without hypnosis. While most underlying states hold positive and pleasant memories, unresolved trauma is normally held in underlying states.

HOW LONG DO EGO STATES LAST?
Can we get rid of an ego state? When we develop an ego state, will we always have it? There is some disagreement about this; Watkins (2000) believes ego states can leave. We can be sure that most ego states last throughout our lives. When speaking directly with ego states, using hypnosis, they reveal a need to continue

existing, and often a fear that the therapist will try to get rid of them. They see their role as useful, and sometime believe the person will die if they do not continue to exist. The best way to help a client who has an ego state that is causing a neurotic response is to help that state change its role, rather than to attempt to get rid of it. Techniques for assisting clients in changing ego state responses are described in Chapter 3.

Occasionally an ego state will say, "It would be better if I leave." and it will appear that the ego state leaves. It is probable that the state is merely becoming inactive. Since some ego states are elusive and some are reluctant to talk it is difficult to determine if a state has actually left.

Ego states will also claim to merge with another state. There is no compelling need to know whether states can leave or merge, since the goal of Ego State Therapy is to reach the goals of the client, not to determine the disposition of states. Related states will sometimes report that a state has left or merged, and while this lends evidence to the notion that states can leave or merge, it is not conclusive evidence. Often states are unaware of the existence of other states.

Conceptually, I view an ego state as a neural pathway that has been formed from intense use. This pathway may be accessed via other ego states (pathways) by lines of communication that may be connected, changed, or disconnected. With this interpretation, it does not make sense that the neural pathway could be erased, but it is conceivable that the pathway may be separated or changed in the connections of communication. It is not unusual for an ego state to be generally unknown by most other states.

IS THERE AN AGE WHEN WE NO LONGER DEVELOP NEW EGO STATES?
Most of our ego states form in early childhood, with the formation of states in adolescence being fewer, but normal. By late adolescence we have gathered an array of ego states that can be applied to almost any life circumstance. After this time we switch into and out of states that are most energized to become executive at any time. A state will continue to evolve, but may have started at a young age. For example, early in school, or even before school, a

"Study" state may begin. This "Study" state may evolve through-out school and adulthood, refining techniques and getting better at its craft. An early "Contemplative" state that may have started when left alone in a boring room in childhood, and may be the same state that ponders the basic constructs of the universe later in life.

It is possible to acquire new states at any time in life. These adult born states are more rare, and some individuals may not develop states in adulthood. Since most states are developed when the person has no existing states to deal with the current situation, adults will only develop a new state when placed in a situation where they are growing in a new way. Examples of this might include John (a man with a traditional male upbringing) developing a nurturing state to raise a baby when he became a sole parent, or Martha (a woman with a traditional female upbringing) developing a rough/tough state when going through basic military training.

WHAT IS EGO STATE COMMUNICATION?
Ego states can be thought of as mini personalities. They are not complete personalities, but each has particular traits. States that often become executive have good lines of communication between each other. There are states that rarely become executive, and they may have poor or no lines of communication with the surface states. It is not unusual for a person to report having little or no memory from a number of years in childhood. Sometimes these individuals fear they may be hiding from some trauma by blocking memories. I have found that normally they have no memory because their life during those years was rather routine, with no major moves or life occurrences. Using Ego State Therapy and hypnosis, an ego state from the lost years may be accessed and introduced to a more surface state with the instruction that they will be able to continue to communicate. After this line of communication is established, memories from childhood will continue to become available to the surface states.

I have a child state that can feel very fragile. It can also truly enjoy a loving hug when it is safe. This child state has a strong line of communication with a fear ego state and my fear ego state has a

9

strong communication with an anger ego state. My child state does not directly communicate with my anger ego state, but if it is threatened my fear state gets the message immediately and may contact my anger state and my anger state responds to the outside world. Before I learned my ego states my intellectual ego state had a knowledge that I was sometimes fragile, but there were no direct lines of communication between my child state and my intellectual state.

States sometimes communicate in clusters. An obsessive-compulsive state (of a past client) communicated well with some ally states, but not at all with most other states. A childhood fearful state would call upon the "Checking" state to create a safe single-mindedness where concerns could be excluded. The "Checking" state that continually checked locks and water faucets or taps was 'hated' by some other states that wanted to get on with life, have a job, and get sleep. She had difficulty maintaining a job, since it took her so long to continually check everything before leaving home, as well as her need to check things at work. Some of her states would say, "I hate myself, I have to check everything all the time. I want to get on with my life." They were saying that they hated the checking state. Although there was an awareness of the existence of each other, there was no line of communication between these states and the "Checking" state. The "Checking" state communicated well with and responded to some fear states that needed the "Checking" state to take over, to escape from trauma they carried. When she was in the checking state it was as though she were in a trance avoiding the pain held by these fearful states. They would feel trauma and call on the "Checking" state to take over. The fear states and checking state made up a cluster of states that communicated together, and she had other states making up other clusters that communicated well together.

My child state, fear state, and anger state are a cluster that communicate together, and my anger state also has lines of communication with some more adult states that may call on it. Ego state mapping (section 3.3.1) allows people to learn about their states, the lines of communication, and the way the states feel about each other.

HOW DO EGO STATES DIFFER FROM MULTIPLE PERSONALITIES?

Many people think 'multiple personality' when they first hear about ego states. There are major differences between Dissociative Identity Disorder or Multiple Personality and ego states (Watkins and Watkins, 1988, 1986). We all have ego states. Multiple Personalities are quite different. They develop in a small minority of cases when a young child experiences extreme abuse continuing over an extended period of time. When some children experience chronic abuse, as an unconscious coping mechanism there is a breakdown of communication between the ego states so the child can experience the next day without memory of the abuse the night before. Some children are able to learn to not remember what happened while in their previous ego state. Over time they can become so proficient at this "not remembering" that the ego states become separated in communication. When this happens, each state has to learn to take on a more full range of roles since it cannot as easily call on other states and retain a memory of what happened while in last state. Persons who are multiple experience periods of blackouts during their day, because often when they switch personalities they have no memory of what they were doing, or why they were doing it, just moments before. While a person with normal ego states may walk from the living room to the kitchen, open the refrigerator and think, "now why did I come in here?" a multiple may open the refrigerator and think, "Why am I here, how long have I been here, where was I before, and what was I doing?" Ego State Therapy is an excellent tool for working with multiples (see section 4.5), but normal ego state function should not be confused with multiple personality.

1.2 Introjects

An introject is a manifestation of a person significant in the life of the client. A five-year-old ego state (of an adult client) may have an introject of 'father' or 'mother' as they were at the time the client was five. A different introject may represent the same parent at a different time. An introject may represent a person as they are currently in the life of the client. For example, there may be an introject of a partner, friend, or parent. Introjects may be of living or dead persons, but they are of persons who are, or have been, meaningful in the life of the client. The client is able to take on the role of an introject and speak with the quality and feelings that the introject represents to the client. The client may be surprised by the feelings that are experienced while an introject is executive. By experiencing an introject in first person the client gains understanding of the introject, the limitations of the introject, and the feelings of the introject, as internalized.

Unlike ego states, introjects may be asked to leave. They do not claim to be part of the person. Introjects can be worked with in much the same way as ego states and inner strength, and they can change. Introjects may be kind and helpful, or may be scary or abusive. If most of the significant people in a person's life were benevolent, then most of that person's introjects will be benevolent. An introject that has been internalized as cold and scary may, through ego state negotiation, become warm and caring. It is often helpful for ego states to be encouraged to express themselves to introjects. If an introject was or is an abuser it is helpful for the client to express true and accurate feelings to the introject. The hypnotherapist can help the client to express feelings to a malevolent introject by being first to speak those feelings, "What you did was wrong!"

Introjects may be easily accessed. Using imagery, when the hypnotized client relates a place where another person is present, the client may be asked to give information about where the other person is and what they are doing. The client may be asked to talk as the other person (the introject). For example, "Is it alright with you if I speak directly with mother?" (Permission given) "I would like you to be your mother now. Mother, I want you to look back and see 'frightened'" (the ego state name the client has given to a child part). "I want to speak directly with you, mother. When you are ready to speak, just say, "I'm ready"." The client will then speak as mother, and will be able to switch back and forth between the ego state and the introject gaining insight, understanding, and expression beneficial to release and empowerment.

1.2.1 Nature of an Introject

- Introjects have the traits of meaningful people who are, or have been, in the life of the client.

- They may be representations of living or dead persons, currently in the life of the client or from a younger age.
- The client is able to allow the introject to become executive. The client is able to speak as the introject.
- Introjects may be kind, indifferent, or malevolent.
- Introjects may be changed, or asked to leave.
- Introjects do not begin as defense mechanisms, and they do not claim to have always been with the client.
- Introjects are present in all persons.

1.3   *Inner Strength*

The "Inner Strength" state (Frederick and McNeal, 1999) has many of the attributes of ego states and is referred to in some literature as an ego state (Watkins, 1993). It may be worked with in the same manner as ego states, although there are definite differences between inner strength and ego states. When asked how old it feels the "Inner Strength" state responds, "Oh, I am the same age as 'name of the client'." When asked when it was born, "I was born with 'name of client'." When asked to name itself the "Inner Strength" state responds with something like, 'inner self', 'spiritual self', 'inner strength', or 'higher self'. Inner strength often asserts it has knowledge relating to the purpose of the individual. Inner strength maintains a consistent role, while the role of ego states may be dramatically changed.

Inner strength may be accessed by first bringing out ego states in a manner described in Chapter 2. Allow the client to become comfortable in moving from one state to another. Next something may be stated like, "There is a strong and clear part that has always been there. It was there when you were born, and it is this part that has ideas about what is important in your life. I would like speak with that inner voice now. When you are ready to speak just say, "I'm here"."

1.3.1 *Nature of Inner Strength*

- Inner strength reports being born with the client.
- Inner strength speaks with a clear, caring, and strong voice.

- Inner strength cannot be removed or changed in nature, although its role can be expanded. It may be asked to help other states, or it may be asked to assign roles to ego states as situations arise.
- Inner strength purports to have a wisdom about the purpose of the individual.
- Inner strength may report having low or high energy. When it has higher energy it may take on a greater role. Over time it may be able to gain strength or energy as other states change in their roles.
- Everyone appears to have an Inner Strength state, although it is occasionally not accessed during the first attempt.

1.4   Ego States and Physiology

It is possible to be relaxed and calm, with muscles loose, breathing and heart beat slow, hands warm. Enter the thought of a prowler outside. Adrenaline is released with the nervous thought. This is the neurotransmitter, epinephrine. The body becomes tense, breathing speeds, digestion slows, and the hands cool as circulation slows with more blood retained in the trunk area of the body. The heart beats faster, eyes dilate, and even the hair stands a bit straighter. Our physical strength temporarily increases to fight or flee. These changes all occur in reaction to a nervous thought in the brain. What happens in our mind impacts on our body.

Internal and underlying ego states also impact our physiology. Studies have revealed that underlying ego states can learn to affect our body in specific ways (e.g., migraine headache), and that they can use this knowledge to meet their needs (Emmerson and Farmer, 1996). John Watkins' first work with ego states was to alleviate psychosomatic symptoms caused by war trauma (Watkins and Watkins, 1981). Ego states holding trauma were causing psychosomatic symptoms. Underlying, traumatized states can cause minor and severe physiological symptoms. Non-traumatized states can use physical symptoms to protect us in a manner they see as appropriate. Resolution of underlying trauma and negotiation with underlying ego states can result in immediate changes in physical symptoms. Ego State Therapy is useful in determining which symptoms may be psychosomatic, and which symptoms are less likely to be, and it can help facilitate a moderation or removal of those symptoms.

1.5   Ego States and Psychology

Our feelings can seem elusive. On a beautiful day we can feel melancholy for no apparent reason. We can react to a person in a manner that is surprising, even to us. A chronic depression can be of unknown origin. Everything has a cause, and the cause is not always known by a surface ego state. Unresolved ego states can lie beneath the surface and express feelings that are yet to be settled. How we feel psychologically is much a result of unresolved issues and of internal ego states that do not cooperate or respect each other. The phrase, "at peace with one's self" really means the parts of the person have resolution to past problems and the parts of the person respect each other. If a person consistently feels bad about what one part says, or does, that person will not feel inner peace. Our ego states affect how we feel psychologically, and Ego State Therapy is a tool that can help facilitate that desired inner peace.

1.6   Beginnings

The development of Ego State Therapy as a unified theory and intervention can be traced to the last quarter of the 20th Century. John and Helen Watkins established the therapy, as it is presently understood. John Watkins developed the theoretical underpinnings necessary for its therapeutic applications. His early work and research helped define the therapy, and Helen Watkins' therapeutic advances and her own theoretical contributions helped broaden Ego State Theory into both a personality theory and a therapy applicable to a wide range of psychological concerns. Paul Federn had been the first to use the term 'ego state' in describing the subsections of the personality, although his theoretical work did not extend to research or therapeutic application.

A complete edition of the *American Journal of Clinical Hypnosis* dedicated to this new intervention in 1993 illustrated the establishment of Ego State Therapy. The Watkins' book, *Ego States: Theory and Therapy* was published in 1997, as the first major text defining the theory.

Ego State Therapy grew from the amalgamation of psychotherapy and hypnosis. During the mid-1970s John and Helen Watkins merged the continually developing fields of psychotherapy and hypnosis to found ego state theory and therapy (Watkins and Watkins, 1981).

By the mid-1970s the psychotherapeutic world was very different from the relative psycho-theoretical void of 1900. John Watkins was able to draw from the works of various therapists and theorists, including those of Paul Federn (1952).

> What is new in Ego State Therapy is its integration of both theoretical concepts and treatment strategies drawn from a wide variety of previous therapies. In one sense it is eclectic, but in still another sense we have developed a fairly distinct theory of personality functioning (J. G. Watkins, 1978a) and an array of treatment procedures around its theoretical position. (Watkins and Watkins, 1981, p. 253)

Watkins had been distilling his own theories for many years. In 1949 he wrote a landmark book pertaining to his hypnotic work with war neuroses (J. G. Watkins, 1949). He was well aware of not only psychotherapeutic theories, but he was well published in the area of hypnosis. It was through his practice of hypnosis that he recognized the presence of differing states, and gained an understanding of the value of working directly with specific states that have need.

John Watkins was Chief Psychologist for the U.S. Army's 5000 bed Welch Convalescent Hospital in Daytona Beach, Florida at a time when a number of World War II veterans suffered with war related neuroses. His first work with ego states was with a patient suffering from a phobia of the dark, who revealed two distinct states referred to as George and Melvin (Watkins and Watkins, 1981). Watkins detailed this case in his book on war neuroses and hypnosis (Watkins, 1949), although at the time he had not sufficiently developed his theory to recognize the states as ego states, thinking them to be multiple personalities (Watkins and Watkins, 1997).

During the 1950s John Watkins became aware of the theories of Paul Federn (1952) and Edorado Weiss (1960). From these theorists came his first understandings of the nature of ego states. He writes, "A personal analysis with training analyst Edorado Weiss (1960), who had himself been analyzed by Paul Federn and trained by Freud, brought acquaintance with Federn's ego state theories..." (Watkins and Watkins, 1997, p. ix). While Freud had seen only three divisions of the psyche, the Id, Ego, and Superego, Federn (1952) had become aware of the ego state structure, and Watkins was able to apply Federn's constructions to his own clients.

By the mid-1970s John Watkins had distilled his work and theories sufficiently to coin the term, Ego State Therapy, and begin writing about the approach as a unified theory (Watkins and Watkins, 1981). Prior to his beginning collaborative work with Helen in 1972, John Watkins had the opportunity to work with a number of dissociative identity disorder (multiple personality) patients, which contributed to his understanding of the dissociative process.

Beginning in 1972, John and Helen Watkins worked together at the University of Montana developing Ego State Therapy (Watkins and Watkins, 1981). It was after the two Watkins begin work together that the true foundations of Ego State Therapy were laid. John Watkins stated

> ... the real significance of the 'separating defense' as being more broadly based throughout a continuum extending from normal personality structure at one end to severely dissociated personalities at the other end did not emerge until collaboration in the early 1970s with my wife and colleague, Helen H. Watkins. (Watkins and Watkins, 1997, p. x)

Helen worked extensively with clients, and developed many strategies and therapy techniques. Her article on the silent abreaction technique (1980) led to her identification with this technique, as the silent abreaction lady (H. H. Watkins, personal communication, December, 1995). John concentrated on intensive treatments and on experimentation involving ego states. Ego state theory was mainly developed from 1973 to 1975, and this period of early development was reflected in the literature in articles, tapes and books (J. G. Watkins, 1976, 1977, 1978a, 1978b; H. H. Watkins, 1978; J. G. Watkins and H. H. Watkins, 1976, 1979a, 1979b, 1979c, 1981).

One of the factors that has prevented a more rapid expansion of Ego State Therapy is that to practice the therapy properly, hypnotic training is necessary and many therapists presently lack such training. Hypnosis is becoming better understood, and an increasing number of training institutions are available. Hypnosis and Ego State Therapy share a symbiotic relationship as the growth of each enhances the growth of the other. As the power and effectiveness of Ego State Therapy becomes better known it will be incumbent upon those responsible for training to ensure that therapists necessarily receive a hypnosis component in their study. Considering the speed psychotherapy and hypnosis developed we can expect that developments in Ego State Therapy will continue over a number of years. The power and efficacy of Ego State Therapy will ensure the continued development of its theory and techniques, and will lead to its greater use and broader acceptance.

1.7   *Efficacy*

Research indicates that Ego State Therapy is effective in assisting clients with both psychological and somatic symptoms. Emmerson and Farmer (1996) found, using a time series experimental investigation of an ego state intervention, that women with menstrual migraine were able to experience not only a reduction in headaches, but also in depression, and anger. Following a four week treatment with Ego State Therapy, their monthly average number of days with migraine went from 12.2 to 2.5, and along with this decline in headaches there was a significant decline in levels of depression and anger. John and Helen Watkins (1997) studied 42 clients who had received Ego State Therapy (median 11 hours) and had also received other types of therapy (median 145 hours). Twenty-four clients said Ego State Therapy met their expectations, while only seven clients said other therapies met their expectations. In a medical study, Ego State Therapy facilitated a patient's complete remission of Reflex Sympathetic Dystrophy, when trauma held by a childhood ego state was processed (Gainer, 1993).

1.8   Related Therapies

There are a number of therapies that share relationships with Ego State Therapy. The following is not considered a complete list of those therapies.

1.8.1   Psychoanalysis

Just as John and Helen Watkins can be viewed as the originators of Ego State Therapy, Sigmund Freud can be thought of as the father of psychotherapy. While many therapists predate Freud, his massive body of work defining his constructions of the personality and his prescriptions of therapeutic interventions laid the foundations for later theoretical and practical development.

Freud saw personality and mental health resulting from the experiences of early childhood. He postulated stages of psychological development and believed that specific psychological adjustments were tied to the nature of developmental training and experiences. One of the enduring tenets of his theories is that early childhood traumas often result in adulthood neuroses. A situational neurosis is a repeated inappropriate response to a particular type of life situation. According to Freud (1901), a person who often responds to a loud criticism by becoming quiet and withdrawn, rather than responding in a situational appropriately fashion, does so because of some early childhood trauma. Freud believed that through psychoanalysis patients could bring the unconscious memory of the trauma to the conscious. This process was viewed as instrumental in the resolution of neuroses.

Ego state theorists accept Freud's contention that previously experienced, unprocessed traumas affect adulthood responses, but they differ greatly from psychoanalysts in the therapeutic interventions for the resolution of the unwanted responses. Psychoanalysts view therapy as a process necessarily involving a number of years, which includes free association, analysis of resistance, dream interpretation, transference, and interpretation of transference. Ego state therapists view therapy as a process of working with traumatized, or needy states, to assist them in processing and becoming empowered. Clients normally experience preferred change quickly.[2]

1.8.2   Gestalt Therapy

Frederick Perls (1969) started Gestalt Therapy during the 1950s borrowing heavily from Jacob Moreno's Psychodrama (Moreno, 1946). Gestalt therapy shares more techniques with Ego State Therapy, than any other major therapy. Gestalt therapists attempt to locate and bring forward the feelings associated with the pre-senting concern, and then process those feelings. Although Gestalt theory does not adequately explain how this technique benefits the client, it is actually an impressive technique to bring to the executive (consciousness) the state that needs facilitation. Gestalt means whole, and gestalt therapists believe if part of the whole is injured (traumatized) in some way, then the whole person cannot function fully. Ego state therapists share this belief. Another Gestalt technique that closely resembles techniques used in Ego State Therapy is the empty chair technique. A Gestalt therapist may ask a client to sit in one chair to explain one aspect of self and sit in another chair to allow another aspect to be explained. Again, the Gestalt therapist is bringing to the executive ego states and working with them. Gestalt theory does not include ego states, or how they were formed, and while the array of gestalt techniques is impressive, these techniques do not include hypnosis. It is hyp-nosis and theory (Emmerson, 1999) that most separates Ego State Therapy from Gestalt Therapy. Hypnosis allows a greater access to ego states, and ego state theory allows a better understanding of the personality so the therapist can best proceed with the most appropriate therapeutic techniques.

1.8.3   Transactional Analysis

The only major therapy that also uses the term ego state is *trans-actional analysis*. Like John Watkins with Ego State Therapy, Eric

---

[2] It is interesting to note that Carl Jung (1970), the founder of Analytic Therapy and a contemporary of Freud, spoke of the multiple subconscious parts of the individual.

Berne (1961) originated the theoretical underpinnings of transactional analysis from the work of Paul Federn (1952). Unlike John Watkins and Paul Federn, Berne theorized only five ego states (two parent states, an adult state, and two child states), and he believed that everyone had the same states. Transactional analysis deals heavily with the ego state communication patterns between persons; e.g., one person's parent state may speak to another person's child state.

Transactional analysis can be viewed as a cognitive training therapy, with clients learning about the five states and learning about how they speak and hear from these states. There is an effort to balance the states so the individual does not operate too heavily within any state. This differs greatly from Ego State Therapy where clients learn about their idiosyncratic states, seek and process trauma, and facilitate improved communication between states within the individual. Ego state theorists believe that no two people have the same states. Ego State Therapy is very much a process therapy, where change occurs through the work that occurs during the hypnosis session. Ego State Therapy helps clients to learn their states, and to gain resolution to trauma. While therapists who use transactional analysis work on communication between the client and others, ego state therapists more often work on communication within the client; communication between states, so the client can feel more settled and less pulled in different directions.

1.8.4 Other Therapies

The three psychotherapies above are directly linked in theory with Ego State Therapy. This presentation does not constitute a complete listing of therapies that share theoretical linkages with Ego State Therapy. Ego state therapists often use techniques from other therapies, and modalities, developed during the last century.

Cognitive behavioral techniques are often used within ego state sessions. After the resolution of a trauma that a state may have held for many years, it is often beneficial to give behavioral 'homework' for the client to gain confidence in a paced fashion.

Family therapy techniques are often used when working with ego states. Working among the states of a client is not unlike working with the members of a family, and positive negotiation skills are useful skills for the ego state therapist. Caul (1984) refers to using internal group therapy techniques for negotiating among the states of an individual.

Voice Dialogue and *Psychosynthesis* are two therapies that appear to resemble Ego State Therapy. Both access ego states and work with them. Neither have the theoretical understanding of the personality structure that ego state theory provides, and neither have techniques developed to find trauma and resolve it, or map an individual's states in the way Ego State Therapy provides. These therapies assume pre-existing defined states while ego state theory holds that no two people will have the same ego state structure.

Voice Dialogue

The following quote illustrates a major difference between voice dialogue and ego state therapies.

> "Therefore, if you have been feeling that you are not expressing yourself fully, or that one part of your personality is dominating your life — maybe your Ambitious Self, your Pleaser or your Lazy Self — you can get in touch with the relevant self and find out why it is acting as it does. When you have a good understanding of it and are no longer completely identified with it, you can access an opposite of that self which has probably been suppressed for a long time and is dying to have a voice". (What is Voice Dialogue? website, 2000)

Ego states do not necessarily have an opposite. They develop according to need and often there is no need to have an opposite of a state.

Psychosynthesis

Psychosynthesis theory holds that we each have the following parts, Sensation, Emotion-Feeling-Impulse Desire, Imagination, Thought, Intuition, Will, and Central point or the personal self

(What is Psychosynthesis? website, 2000). An interesting aspect of both voice dialogue and psychosynthesis is that they, and a number of other therapies, attempt to identify and deal with separate parts of the personality. While they may not be as developed as Ego State Therapy in terms of, research, theory, and techniques, ego states have been identified, and the value of working with them has been understood. Voice dialogue and psychosynthesis may be thought to occupy the theoretical middle ground between transactional analysis and Ego State Therapy. Transactional analysts assume we have only five predetermined states, voice dialogue and psychosynthesis theorists assume we have many relatively predetermined states, and ego state theorists assume we each have many states that distinctly make up our ego state map; our internal family of states.

Chapter 2

Accessing Ego States in Therapy

How can the therapist learn to access and speak with the different ego states that exist within the individual? Imagine a classroom full of students. The students on the front row are awake and attentive, some more than others. Other students in the room often do not pay attention to what goes on in the room, but the students in the front row see and remember most things. The rest of the students in the room are paying varying degrees of attention. Some are in a sound sleep. Others are whispering in small groups. And some are watching what is going on at the front of the classroom. Occasionally one may act on a need and make a disturbance in the classroom. There may be a student hanging onto a lot of pain and turmoil, an unstable student ready to erupt. There is one rule in the classroom that the students honor. Only one student is able to talk at once.

The students are all different and all have different problems and talents. Some of them talk often, and some that have a lot to say, some talk very seldom. Some are afraid to talk, even thinking they may be asked to leave the room. Some students do not like each other, and often argue. Every classroom is made up of a different set of students. Each classroom has it own personality.

At the front of the room, standing next to the blackboard is the teacher. The teacher is visually blind. Although she has been in several classrooms before, she has never really known where she was. She has thought she was there to tutor a single student. When she talks, it is the students in the front row that usually listen and respond to her. Even though the voices of the different students sound different, the teacher has not paid much attention to that.

Of course, the classroom represents the family of ego states of a single person. The students on the front row are the surface ego states, those that most often become executive, those that maintain a good memory of the daily activities. The rest of the students represent the underlying ego states. The teacher is the therapist.

If the teacher talks to the class thinking that she is speaking to a single student, then the member of the class who really needs the help of the teacher may not even be listening. The student in the back of the room who carries pain may continue to feel neglected and unheard. Students who argue with each other, and those who do not like each other continue to make the classroom an uncomfortable place for all students. The students with specific talents may not be able to use them when the right time arises.

The question is, how can the blind teacher learn to recognize the students, draw them out, attend to their needs, help the group work together, and discover which students have special talents? How can the therapist learn to access and speak with the different ego states of the individual?

There are both non-hypnotic and hypnotic methods to access ego states. The non-hypnotic methods give access only to the surface states. In the classroom example, they give access only to the students on the front row. Recognizing the surface states (students on the front row) and talking with them individually gives more power in therapy than treating them as a single state.

Hypnotic access of ego states allows the therapist to work with both surface and underlying states. Often the client's problems stem from underlying states, and it is only through hypnotic access that direct and efficient problem resolution can be achieved. Just as an angry child in the back of the classroom can affect the mood of the class, an underlying ego state can require direct attention and resolution for the client to feel peace.

It is important to note that every therapist already accesses ego states, whether or not it is consciously recognized. Any time we are conscious, an ego state is executive. When the client sits down and begins talking, it is one of that client's ego states that is talking. The problem is that the state that is talking my not be the best state for therapeutic intervention. Talking with a rational, head state may allow the therapist to easily find an ally that is against the obsessive compulsive checking, an ally that wants the anger management client to be rational, or that wants the smoker to stop smoking. Ego State Therapy is about learning to access ego states, to talk directly with the state or states where intervention is most useful.

2.1 Non-Hypnotic Access

Non-hypnotic access of ego states is appropriate for therapists who are not trained in hypnosis, or who are not ready to work with hypnosis. It may also be useful for working with clients who are not able to consider a hypnotic intervention. Two methods of non-hypnotic access are presented in sections 2.1.1 and 2.1.2. The therapist who is familiar with ego states will often be able to recognize when the client changes states, even without using an access method. The informed therapist will be able to work cognizantly with ego states, gaining an awareness of when a different state becomes executive, and gaining an awareness of individual ego state needs.

2.1.1 Empty Chair Technique

One of the easiest ways to access ego states is the *empty chair technique*. Some therapists who are unaware of ego state theory use this technique, or a version of it. Gestalt therapists often use a two chair variety of this technique, so two ego states can communicate, or so an ego state can communicate with an introject (see sections 1.2 and 1.8.2).

Consider the example of Matthew from the beginning of Chapter 1. He sees Emma playing with a child, and he feels and believes, "This is the woman for me. I love her and want to spend the rest of my life with her." Later in the same day she criticizes him about his job as a plumber. He feels defensive and feels and thinks, "What did I ever see in this woman? How can I get out of this relationship?" At least two of Matthew's ego states are disagreeing. He is experiencing internal turmoil, internal ego state argument.

The therapist can place two chairs in front of Matthew. In order to illustrate this technique the following example is presented:

> **Therapist**: Matthew, I'm hearing that part of you wants to marry your partner, and part of you doesn't. It would be really helpful for me to be able to hear exactly what each of those parts wants. (The therapist places two chairs in front of Matthew.) When you sit in the chair on the left I want you to tell me only the good things about getting married to Emma. I don't want you to tell me about any reservations you might have. Then when I ask you to sit in the chair on the right, I want you to tell me only the bad things about your getting married to Emma. Nothing but reasons you should not marry her. Do you understand?

When they first hear about this technique, therapists seem to have more fear about it than clients do. Many therapists first think their clients will think it is silly, or will not cooperate. If it is presented professionally, and in a straightforward fashion there should be no problems. I have never had a client who, when offered it, did not participate, and clients find it very useful.

The next step, after answering any questions, is:

> **Therapist**: All right, go ahead and sit in the chair on the left. Now tell me why you want to marry Emma. Tell me only the positive side of getting married to her.

Matthew should be encouraged to continue with reasons to get married. If he starts to inject a reason why he shouldn't (a 'but'), then the therapist needs to stop him immediately, and remind him that while in that chair he should only describe the reasons he wants to marry Emma.

When he finishes with 'pros' then the therapist can continue in the following manner:

> **Therapist**: OK, now I want you to sit in the chair on the right, and when you do tell me only the reasons you do not want to marry Emma.

Again, Matthew is encouraged to relate only the aspects that are against his getting married to Emma. When he has been able to do this, the 'cons' side can be asked to respond to the 'pros' side. It is good to give each ego state a name so they can more easily be identified and called upon with questions.

> **Therapist:** Thanks Matthew. Is it OK if I call you in the right side "Con" and you in the left chair "Pro" for the Con and Pro reasons you are expressing?
>
> **Matthew: Yes.**
>
> **Therapist:** Good. Now, just move to the Pro chair for a minute. Pro, did you hear what Con said about marrying Emma?
>
> **Matthew: Yes.**
>
> **Therapist:** Tell Con what you think about what he said. Just tell him exactly what you think.

Matthew is encouraged to continue switching between the chairs allowing the two ego states to discuss the issue. Occasionally, Matthew can be asked to sit back in the original chair, where he can be given feedback, and asked other questions. An example of this is:

> **Therapist:** Matthew, just watching that conversation, I noticed when Pro was talking you were more animated, more excited about what you were saying about your future. When Con was talking it seemed like you had more fear about what she thinks about you now. I did not hear anything about your future. Can you comment on that?

Or:

> **Therapist:** Matthew, I hear Pro saying … and Con saying … Can you see a way they may be able to come to some agreement? What does each need?

Working with this technique, it is not unusual for a third ego state to emerge, with different thoughts and feelings. You can continue to add chairs to accommodate additional states that have an interest in the decision.

This is an example of ego states talking with each other directly. It is also possible to provide a chair for Emma. When Matthew sits in the Emma chair, he is instructed to be Emma and say and feel the things she would say and feel. When he does this he is speaking as an introject (see section 1.2).

29

> **Therapist:** Matthew, you know Emma very well. You know how she responds. When you sit in this chair I want you to be Emma. I want you to allow yourself to feel her feelings and respond as Emma.

This allows Matthew's introject of Emma a chance to talk with his ego states. It is a very useful technique that can allow the client to get a better perspective of what is possible in a relationship, and a better perspective of how another person may feel. It can help a client understand the boundaries of what is possible in a relationship. The introject can be of a living or dead person. It can be of a person as they are now, or as they were at a time in the past.

2.1.2   Conversational Technique

A second technique for accessing ego states without hypnosis is the *conversational technique*. This is a simple process and may be undertaken at any time during therapy. A therapist who has not planned to use Ego State Therapy in a particular session may elect to use the conversational technique when the client begins talking about his or her different parts. Client statements such as, "part of me wants to go to school, and part of me doesn't", or "sometimes I love him, and sometimes I can't stand being near him" can be viewed as an expressed need for resolution of the internal conflict. It is not good enough to merely continue talking about these ego states that are in conflict. They deserve to be directly heard and to have the opportunity to achieve an internal resolution. Of course, hypnotic Ego State Therapy may be used at this time, but if the therapist or the client are not ready for hypnosis (most often it is the therapist) then this non-hypnotic technique may be used.

The conversational technique is similar to the empty chair technique, without the use of different chairs. The following steps are involved in this technique (listed first, and then explained):

1. The therapist becomes aware of at least two parts of the person that are in conflict or the therapist becomes aware of different parts with different needs.
2. The therapist speaks to the client in a manner that brings to the executive the part that it will be most helpful to speak with at the time.

3. The therapist asks to speak with only one part at a time.
4. The therapist speaks with the client in such a manner to bring to the executive a different part that will be most helpful to speak with at the time.
5. The therapist asks to speak with only the second part.
6. The therapist may ask to speak with other parts or may alternate between the parts already spoken with in order to reach a resolution.

Explanation:

1. *The therapist becomes aware of at least two parts of the person that are in conflict or the therapist becomes aware of different parts with different needs.*
    "I constantly give in to people and say I will do what they want, then later I resent having to do it." Here one part likes to please and will give in without properly communicating with other parts that will have to deal with the consequences.

    "I come home from work and I go straight to the fridge and eat. Later I am disappointed about what I have done." Here one part is attempting to satisfy a need with food, without properly communicating with other parts that do not like the eating pattern.

    While many of the issues uncovered with the conversational technique may be dealt with without hypnosis, when the issues are tied to underlying states and traumas from the past, an ego state hypnotic intervention would be a preferred manner of resolution. Underlying states be accessed with the use of hypnosis.

2. *The therapist speaks to the client in a manner that brings to the executive the part that it will be most helpful to speak with at the time.*
    This can occur in normal conversation without giving the client any specific instructions. If an issue for a client is that her mother consistently pressures her to have a child, and this makes the client angry and reactionary toward her mother, the following type statements and questions might be used to

31

bring the angry ego state to the executive. Of course, they would be woven into the conversation with the client.

> "Your mother sounds like she would really like a grandchild. How does her pressing this point make you feel? It appears that your mother sometimes does not hear you on this issue. That must be frustrating. When you are sitting in the living room with your mother and she warns you about waiting too long to have a child and tells you how much joy they bring to your life, what happens inside you? How does that part of you that wishes she would leave you alone feel?"

3. *The therapist asks to speak with only one part at a time.*
    After the client exhibits the reaction and body language revealing the preferred part is executive, it is good to let the client know that you want to continue talking just with that part for a while. This gives the client clarity about what is expected. The client will be able to cooperate and help ensure that the executive ego state remains executive, and another ego state does not jump in with a different perspective. An example of this request is, "I would like to talk only with this part of you that is really angry with you mother. I only want to hear from the angry part right now. I want to hear what this part has to say. Later I will want to hear from the other parts that have different feelings."

    It is sometimes the case that even after making this request that an ego state with a different opinion spontaneously comes to the executive. When this happens it should be noted and another request to be able to hear the desired ego state can be made. For example, if the client starts talking about how nice 'mother' really is, the therapist can say something like, "I think I am hearing a different part. The part I was talking with was still angry. I will want to hear what all parts have to say, but right now I would like to talk only with that part that is angry with your mother."

4. *The therapist speaks with the client in such a manner to bring to the executive a different part that will be most helpful to speak with at the time.*
    Suppose the client has the concern of being frustrated with her mother because on the one hand the client is angry about the pressure from her mother to have a child, and on the other hand she loves and respects her mother and wants to please

her and make her happy. After hearing what the angry part has to say, it is appropriate to see what the part that loves and respects her mother has to say. This is assuming that the client has already provided information that leads the therapist to believe that she does love and respect her mother. (Remember, this is very different than talking to an intellectual part that can tell about the disagreements within. It is much more powerful to deal directly with the parts in conflict.) The therapist may say something to the effect of, "Thank you for letting me hear about the anger that is sometimes present concerning the pressure you mother places on you. Now I would like to hear about some of the positive feelings you have toward your mother. You have said she is a great friend for you. What sort of things does she do that allows you to see her as a great friend?"

When the client articulates positive things about her mother she will move from the state that holds resentment and anger and to a state that is proud of her mother. In other words, the state that is proud of her mother will come to the executive.

5.   *The therapist asks to speak with only the second part.*
     Here again, after the client exhibits the verbal/emotional reaction and body language revealing the preferred part is executive, it is good to let the client know that you want to continue talking just with that part for a while. "For a little while, I would just like to talk with this part of you that is quite positive about your mother." It is important to hear each part well. Sometimes a part rarely has an opportunity to express itself without another part breaking into the executive. For example, previously the client may not have been able to completely express her anger toward her mother, because each time the angry part came to the executive the part that felt positive toward her mother may have felt guilty and felt a need to say something nice about her mother. The angry part would have been cut short by the other part taking over the executive. If the parts are to reach a resolution, and if the client is to have internal peace, each part needs to be able to express itself completely. This allows not only the therapist to hear, but it also allows the other ego states of the client to hear and get a better internal understanding.

6. *The therapist may ask to speak with other parts or may alternate between the parts already spoken with in order to reach a resolution.* Negotiation is necessary for the different parts to reach a resolution. You can ask one part what it would like to say to another. For example, the mother positive part may be asked what it would like to say about 'mother' to the angry part.

Therapist: I can hear that you have a lot of respect for your mother. At the same time I can hear that part of you is quite angry with her for her consistently pressuring you to have a baby. What would this part of you that loves your mother like to say to the part of you that is angry at her? What might be helpful for that part to hear?

Client: I guess I would say that she means well. She sees herself missing out on being able to enjoy a grandchild, and it is important to her.

Therapist: And I am wondering how the part that has been angry with your mother hears that. What would the part that has been angry like to say back?

Client: She just needs to learn that this is my life and I am not her. She had her life, and now it is my turn. If I decide to have a child that will be one thing, but even if I never have one she should leave me alone.

Therapist: And did this angry part hear the positive part try to explain your mother? What do you think of her just wanting a grandchild?

Client: I know she does, but she needs to leave me alone.

Therapist: Are you able to tell you mother this without getting into an argument?

Client: No. I usually don't say anything until I get pretty upset and then I say too much.

Therapist: It sounds like you need to express yourself in a way that you can feel heard without feeling like you say too much.

Client: I would love to be able to do that.

Therapist: I wonder if you could internally ask the part of you that loves and respects your mother to express to her your real feelings about needing to have the space to make your own decisions regarding having a child. It will be important that all your feelings are expressed to your mother, and if the part of you that loves and respects her tells her, she may be able to hear it. I want to ask you to do something internally, without speaking out loud. Without saying anything out loud, right now I would like the part of you that is angry at your mother to ask the part that is positive toward your mother if it will convey to her your real feelings about having a child. I will give you a moment to do this. (PAUSE) How did it go?

Client: I think it will work. I think my mother may be able to hear me if I tell her in the right way.

This is an example of using the conversational technique for helping internal parts that can benefit from better cooperation and communication. It can result in ego states achieving both more internal respect for each other, and in ego states relating in a more beneficial way to the outside world. It allows ego states to get the direct attention they need. In this example the client could have also been asked to assume the identity of her mother and add that voice to the discussion. This would have been using the mother introject to give the client a better understanding of the whole dynamic between her mother, her love and respect for her mother, and her desire for her own independence.

The conversational technique may also be used to help an ego state that feels a need to achieve to fulfill that need by getting help from other states that have the necessary talents. For a more detailed discussion of techniques that may be used in this regard see section 3.1.4, 'Gaining help from other ego states'.

2.2   *Hypnotic Access*

While the non-hypnotic techniques are useful and can generate excellent growth in therapy, they are not as powerful as the hypnotic techniques for accessing ego states. For example, using the non-hypnotic techniques outlined above Matthew may be able to come to a more clear understanding about marrying Emma. He may be able to gain insights into the relationship, and he may be able to function in a more healthy fashion in the relationship.

He will not be able to discover why he over-reacts defensively when Emma criticizes him. He will not be able to access the underlying child ego state that experienced trauma, and continues to hold that trauma. Hypnosis is needed to allow those ego states to come to the executive and get their needs met.

Let's go back to the metaphor of the classroom as the personality, and the students in the classroom are the ego states. Hypnosis allows the teacher (therapist) to get the attention of the entire room of students, not just those on the front row (the surface states). Hypnosis allows a connection between the problem and the cause of the problem. If we think of Matthew's personality as being his classroom of ego states, his exaggerated response to criticism was caused by an upset state in the back of his ego state classroom. Until that part of Matthew gains a resolution he will continue to respond in a similar, inappropriate fashion to criticism.

It should be noted that it is not unusual for spontaneous hypnosis to occur during a non-hypnotic procedure for accessing ego states. This is due to the focusing during the ego state accessing procedure, even without any formal induction. When this occurs, more ego states are accessible.

2.2.1 Hypnosis

The reader should refer to other texts and training for detail concerning hypnosis, hypnotic inductions, and hypnotic procedures. It is important to note here that among other characteristics of hypnosis is the increased internal focus and internal awareness it provides.

Hypnosis and Ego State Therapy share a symbiotic relationship, as each is enhanced by the other. Without hypnosis, Ego State Therapy provides good theory and technique, but fails to provide access to the full range of states. Without hypnosis, much of the work with ego states could not be accomplished. Ego State Therapy also provides an excellent usage for hypnosis. More therapists will become trained in hypnosis as they discover how useful the tool of hypnosis is when applied in conjunction with Ego State Therapy.

2.2.2   *General Guidelines for Talking with Ego States*

When ego states are accessed it is important to understand some general guidelines in how they may best be addressed. Prior to learning to access ego states hypnotically one should be aware of these guidelines and some useful statements and questions. Using our metaphor from the beginning of this chapter, 'don't walk into the classroom before you have some ideas about how to address the students'.

Below are some useful dialogue and guidelines for working with ego states. Do not use this text verbatim. Always respond spontaneously when speaking with ego states.

The examples of dialogue for good Ego State Therapy are first listed and then each example is explained.

- What can I call you?
- What is your function?
- How old do you feel, or how old was (client) when you came to be?
- What do you need?
- What other parts do you know?
- I would like to talk with a part that would like to help.
- Say, "I'm here", when you are ready.
- I wonder how much you can increase the experience you are having?
- Go to the time when you were "the age felt" and you first had this feeling.
- Are you inside or outside?
- Are you along or with someone else?
- Tell me exactly what is happening.
- I want you to know that this is only a memory.
- Say what you want to say.
- Would you like me to tell him (or her) first?
- Can you ask for a hug?
- What is happening now?
- Is it OK with you if I talk with the other part?
- Thank you for speaking with me.
- Is there any part that has a need to say something before we stop for today?

Explanation:

- *What can I call you?*
  When you speak with an ego state it is very important to get a name for that state so you will be able to call upon it again, and the state will know you are calling it to come to the executive to talk. It is also important to have a name so you will be able to ask other states about it.

  States sometimes name themselves according to their role. An intellectual state may give itself the name "Head". States may spontaneously give a name such as Andy or Amy. I normally accept the name that is given without question.

  States can be renamed after therapy has progressed, and I recommend this when negative names are given by the client, such as "Afraid" or "Destroyer". When "Afraid" has resolved the fear I will ask if it would still like to be called "Afraid", or to choose a new name that better fits its feelings. States will usually choose a new name.

  When asking an ego state what it can be called, the client sometimes has difficulty deciding on a name. You can negotiate with the client about what would be a good name for that state. The name for an ego state should always come from that state. Don't accept a name for a state suggested by a different state unless it agrees with this name. For, example one state may see another state as 'Trouble', but that state may not see itself as 'Trouble' and would not like answering to that name.

  It is important to take good notes with the ego state names. Make sure all names are noted along with their roles, strengths, and weaknesses. When a state reveals information concerning other states make notes on the relationship between the states. Some states depend on each other and work closely together, and some states are disliked by other states and thought of as negative.

- *What is your function?*
  Other phrasings of this question are, "What do you do?" or "What is your role?" It is important to note the function of each

state so you can call on that state if it is needed. For example, a state may say its function is to protect, by being brash and defending the person in an argument. This state might be called upon to help a person be more appropriately assertive. When you know this state exists, you will be able to call on it and ask it if it would like to help in this way.

Sometimes the function of a state may be detrimental to the client, for example, the state with a function to give the person a migraine when she gets "too emotional". By learning the function of a state negotiation can alter the function so the negative role can be changed to a positive role, or decreased. A state with a negative function may be told it is a powerful and important state, and that it can help to assist the client in a positive way, a way that will both help the client and gain the state the respect of the other states.

- *How old do you feel, or how old was (client) when you came to be?* The answer to this question normally reveals the age of the client when the ego state you are speaking with first started. When a client is showing a high level of emotion, asking the question, "How old do you feel right now?" is a good first step in discovering the original trauma that causes the emotion.

  It is not unusual for a state to say it does not know how old it feels, or that it feels older than the client. Normally, when the state is experiencing a high level of emotion when the question is asked, a rather young age is given. If the state states it does not know how old it feels, that it feels the age of the client, or that it feels older than the client, I normally proceed to a different line of inquiry, rather than asking the state to go directly to the age it feels.

  States that say they feel older than the client often are states that describe feeling very tired. If a state claims to be from a "Past Life" it can still be worked with to release trauma using the same techniques discussed in Chapter 3 of this book.

- *What do you need?* This is a very good and extremely useful question. When a state seems distressed in any way, you can ask it what it needs, or "What would make you feel better?" If a state says it needs a hug, you can ask to speak with a state that would like to help this state by giving it a hug. If it is afraid, you can ask what it is afraid of, so it can face the fear (for example, tell a perpetrator to go away), and then get the needed help (for example, from another ego state that has the needed strengths). Examples of how states can be helpful include giving nurturing to states that have felt over-exposed, or providing assertive release for states that hold on to frustration and are afraid to say what they feel.

- *What other parts do you know?*
  This is a good question either for ego state mapping, or to build a base of information that may be used in therapy. It helps the therapist understand the internal dynamics of the client, and provides information about states that may be asked to help with a particular function or problem. States that already know each other and help each other are often quickly willing to be helpful in therapy.

- *I would like to talk with a part that would like to help.*
  When a need is found, there is a great resource to meet that need within the client. We each have a variety of ego states. Consider a state that is young, and crying, and feeling alone. The statement, "I would like to talk with a part that would like to help" calls for a state that is not only willing to help, but that wants to help. It is not enough to get a state that is willing to help, since a state that does not really want to participate in a role will not do it for very long. A state that wants to help will normally continue helping.

  To nurture a frightened child state, it is important to find a state that enjoys nurturing. If a strong state that does not enjoy nurturing volunteers to help, that state can be warmly thanked for offering, and told that you really need to talk with a state that would enjoy helping. "I need to speak with a state that cares about children and would really enjoy staying with this child state." It is important that the helping state wants to help and would enjoy helping, rather than merely agreeing to help. A state that wants to help will continue to help far into the future. A state that sees helping as a difficulty will often stop helping in the short-term.

- *Say, "I'm here", when you are ready.*
  When calling on a state that you would like to speak with, it is important to give a clear understanding of how that state is to respond. Without this, the state may not become overtly verbal. After saying, "I would like to talk with a part that..." the state becomes aware that you want to talk with it. The next step is to inform the state how to respond when it is ready to speak. After the state responds with, "I'm here" a conversation may ensue.

- *On a scale of 1 to 100, what is your experience of the feeling you are having?*
  This is not an exact phrasing of this statement, since it needs to be stated in accordance with the experience the client is having. When clients experience anxiety, either as an emotional disturbance or through a physical experience (such as feeling tight around the throat), it is important that they be able to become involved in the experience, in order to locate the origin of the disturbance. Before attempting to discover the origin of a disturbance it is important that the client show significant affect. If considerable affect is shown already, the above question and the one below are not necessary. If considerable affect is not shown, ask the question above, and then follow it with the question below. The question above might be phrased for a particular client, "On a scale of 1 to 100, how much are you experiencing that tightness in the throat right now?"

- *I wonder how much you can increase the experience you are having?*
  This question might be phrased for the client above who indicates an experience level of 70 on the scale, "That's good. I wonder how much you can increase that feeling of tightness in the throat above 70 (pause). What is it now?" This line of questioning is continued until significant affect is demonstrated.

- *Go to the time when you were "the age felt" and you first had this feeling.*
  When the client demonstrates significant affect the, "How old do you feel right now, with that tightness in the throat?" question is

41

appropriate. If the client reports feeling about seven, say, "Go to the time when you were about seven feeling this tightness in the throat for the first time." This takes the client to the origin of the problem. It may still be important to help the client become clear about what is happening, so follow the questions below.

- *Are you inside or outside a building?*
  Immediately following the question above ask, "Are you inside or outside?" The client will normally have an awareness of being inside or outside. This helps the client focus in on the disturbance without giving any suggestions. Then go to the next question.

- *Are you alone or with someone else?*
  This question further facilitates the client to zero in on the original disturbance. After asking this question it is common that the client may be quite emotional. It is imperative that the client be allowed to be in this emotion so it may be resolved. It is the hypnotherapist's duty to allow this emotion to be expressed, regardless of the level of affect. If you feel you are not able to be with a client who is experiencing severe affect, do not begin this line of questioning. It is better not to revisit a trauma, if the trauma is not going to be processed to a positive conclusion.

- *Tell me exactly what is happening.*
  The client is now able to describe, in detail, what happened that started the situational neurosis. It is imperative that the client continues to stay in the ego state at the time that it was traumatized. This is a good time to ask this state what you can call it. You will want to be able to recall that state it at a later time.

- *I want you to know that this is only a memory.*
  Ego states that have experienced trauma may become distressed when relating that trauma. They often exhibit real fear and severe affect. It is important that they be able to remain at the time they were traumatized in order for the fear to be relieved. Still, there are a number of ways that this severe affect can be moderated while resolution is in progress. One statement that can be helpful to a client at this time is, "I want

you to know that this is only a memory. This is not really happening right now." The traumatized state can hear and understand this.

Other statements that can be helpful at this time are, "I am here with you, and I am not going to let anything hurt you", and/or "There is a thick glass wall between you and 'whoever the antagonist is' and you can say absolutely anything you want." I often ask if it is all right if I touch the client's elbow to give the knowledge that I am there for support. The elbow is a non-threatening place to touch, and laying two fingers on the elbow can assure the client that an ally is present. Whenever the need is felt thereafter I will say, "I'm here with you and I'm not going to let anything hurt you" as I temporarily press a bit more on the elbow. I would not touch the elbow without first asking the client for permission.

- *Say what you want to say.*
  It is very important for an ego state to feel expressed. If it holds fear of a threatening introject, it will hold that fear until it is overcome, then it is no longer afraid. By telling an introject what is felt, courage replaces fear. States should be encouraged to say what they feel. They should not be told what to feel, although it is often obvious what is being felt. For example, a state that is showing fear, especially a state that has said to the therapist, "I'm afraid to tell him" is obviously afraid and does not like being frightened.

- *Would you like me to tell him (or her) first?*
  Sometimes a state is too frightened to be able to speak to the aggressive introject. I offer to speak first when this is the case. What I say depends on how the client has described the situation to me. Before speaking directly to the introject, you should ask the client if this is alright, "You can tell him. Do you want me to tell him first?" When speaking directly to the introject speak loudly. Show the client that you are not afraid. Speak punitively, **"You had no right to do what you did!!"**, then to the client, **"OK, now you can tell him. Tell him what you want to tell him!"**

This type of encouragement to express needs should continue until the client has expressed feelings. It is good to ask the client what he or she would like to happen. A common response is a preference for the introject to leave. If this is the case, the client should be encouraged to demand the introject to leave. Continue to check on what happened, "What is happening now?"

When the ego state is expressed, ask again the question, "What do you need now?" Any additional needs can normally be met by calling for other ego states that would like to satisfy the needs of this state on a continuing basis. Here you may ask the question, "I would like to talk with a part that would like to help by..." (See above).

- *Can you ask for a hug?*
  After finding a state that would like to help, a common question to ask the weaker state is, "Can you ask 'name of helping state' for a hug?" Then, after a pause, again asked the question, "What is happening now?" The response is normally very positive. Of course, asking this question will depend on the needs of the troubled state. Each situation should be addressed in relation to the needs at the moment, not in any verbatim fashion.

- *What is happening now?*
  This is an excellent question that may be used at various times with Ego State Therapy. Ego State Therapy allows the therapist to meet the needs of the client; more specifically to meet the needs of ego states that can benefit from resolution. In order to know what needs exist, it is important to stay aware of what the client is experiencing. The progress of the therapy should be directed according to client needs, not directed according to analytical hunches the therapist might have. "Exactly, what is happening now?" is a question that keeps the therapist abreast of progress. Depending on the response, therapy may be directed.

The two most common uses of this question are during the exploration for the origin of the problem, and during the resolution of the problem. By asking a client who is experiencing exactly what is happening, information is gathered that can be used to form the questions to increase the intensity of the feeling so it may be used to go to the origin of the problem (see "On a scale of 1 to 100, what is your experience of the feeling you are having?" above). By asking an ego state that is at the origin of the problem (usually experiencing trauma), "Exactly, what is happening now?" the therapist can determine what resources to call upon to assist with the resolution.

- *Is it OK with you if I talk with the other part?*
  Remember to always get the name of each state you speak with. This allows you to call upon that ego state again when it is useful. Here is an example of the usage of this question. Suppose I am speaking with a seven-year-old child state named 'Small One' and I want to talk with an adult nurturing state called, 'Nurturer'. I might say to the child state, "Thank you for talking with me. I may want to talk with you some more later. Is it OK with you if I talk with 'Nurturer' now?

  This fosters a feeling of trust and respect and facilitates a working relationship. The child state, 'Small One' will be more likely to want to cooperate with therapy and will be more ready to talk again the next time if it is treated with respect. When I finish a therapy session, I glance at my notes and say thank you, by name, to all the states I have spoken with during the session, and I remind them of any work or agreements they have completed.

- *Thank you for speaking with me.*
  As the last question, this question fosters a feeling of trust and respect and facilitates a positive working relationship. See comments above.

- *Is there any part that has a need to say something before we stop for today?*
  It is important to check to see if a part has been left feeling exposed or uneasy because of anything that has happened during the session. If a part is uncomfortable with what has occurred during a session the client may later feel exposed or uneasy, either immediately after the session or within a few hours. By checking if all parts are comfortable with any changes or realignments the client will better be able to experience positive feelings between sessions.

The following guidelines for good Ego State Therapy are listed, and then explained.

- Speak to each state as a person, directly, and do not assume the gender of a state before being told.
- Pay attention to spontaneous switching of states, and show recognition to the newly executive state.
- Always speak respectfully to ego states.
- Always speak respectfully about other ego states when talking with any state.
- Promote an internal dialogue, getting stronger states to help weaker ones.
- Encourage states to trade or change functions, when helpful.
- Map the ego states, and keep track of which ones can communicate with each other, and what the roles of each are. You can later call on ego states you know for help.

Explanation:

- *Speak to each state as a person, directly, and do not assume the gender of a state before being told.*
  If you are speaking with a state called 'Nurturer' phrase sentences such as, "What is your role? How old do you feel, right now? What do you think about that, Nurturer?" Do not phrase sentences where you are not talking directly to the state, "What does Nurturer do? How old does Nurturer feel? What does Nurturer think about that?" Using these statements would encourage a state other than Nurturer to assume the executive and answer.

  It is important that states feel attended to. They may not talk with you unless you talk with them, directly. Be interested in what they have to say, always pay respect, and speak in the way you would like to be spoken to.

  It is not common, but not very unusual for a client to have one or more states of the opposite gender of the client. Therefore, do not assume the gender of a state. Normally you do not need to be concerned with the gender. A male may have an intuitive state that reports itself as female, or a female may have a highly assertive state that reports itself as male. This is not an issue, other than learning to use terms such as 'he' and 'she' appropriately for each state.

• *Pay attention to spontaneous switching of states, and show recognition to the newly executive state.*
  We often change from one ego state to another. This switching occurs spontaneously, not only during our daily routine, but also during therapy. It is helpful to learn to recognize this spontaneous switching in therapy, and it is not difficult to do after gaining some experience in working with ego states. Pay close attention to the presentation level of affect (emotional presentation) and intellectual orientation. Be aware of any nervousness, fear, will, and tone exhibited by the client. A noticeable shift may mean there has been a change in states.

It is possible to notice the shift in individuals even outside of therapy, but when this shift is noticed while actively working with ego states during therapy, normally, the new state should be acknowledged. This can be accomplished with a statement like, "This isn't the Nurturer that is talking now, is it? This seems to be a more reflective state." The client will usually respond with a statement like, "No, I guess it's not." Then it is good to ask for a name for the state you are talking with, and attend to the need it has to be executive.

Often, after attending to the needs of the new state, you will want to return to the state that you were talking with before the shift. This can be accomplished in the following fashion. "Thank you for talking with me. I may want to talk with you more later, but right now I would like to talk with 'Nurturer'. Just say 'I'm here", when you are ready to talk."

Although spontaneous switching can occur during anytime in Ego State Therapy, it most often occurs during the early stages of the session, especially during the first session that ego states are worked with. Continuing to respond to the specific state that is executive helps the ego state to become more aware and involved. There is less spontaneous switching as the session continues, as hypnotic depth deepens and underlying states come to the executive.

- *Always speak respectfully to ego states.*

  It is very important to speak to states respectfully. An important asset the therapist has in promoting resolution and change is the cooperation ego states. It is important that states cooperate with the therapist and with each other. Some states will be afraid to speak, at first, sometimes even fearing that the therapist will try to get rid of them. If a state gains a positive impression about the therapist it will be more eager to be helpful during therapy. Do not make statements like, "You are really difficult, aren't you?" or "You should not do what you are doing." Find ways to pay respect to all states.

  Consider a state that is instrumental in giving a client migraine headaches. It would be detrimental to say, "She does not need you. She would be better off without you." This approach would probably result in the state refusing to talk with you, and might result in the state hiding, and pretending it is not there. It could fear that you might try to make it go away (something that you could not do). It would most likely not result in any change in the role the state has taken on, to give the client migraines.

  An alternative, and preferred approach would be as follows, "I can see you are a very strong state. I know that you came about to help this person. I need your help now to help this person." You can say, "I don't know if you know it, but some of the things you have been doing actually hurt this person, and make some of her other parts wish you were not here. I need your help, and it would be really nice if you could help in a way that would cause the other states to appreciate and like you."

  All states initially were developed to protect or benefit the individual. It can be helpful to remind a state of its original purpose (to help) and respectfully ask for help now for the client. States that have become opposed by other states normally, at first, resist change, and pretend to not care what other states think, or feel, about them. This resistant, obstinate front almost always dissipates with negotiation (see section 3.2.3). When states learn cooperative roles they appear happier in their new roles. The affect change that they show, from 'cold detachment' to 'appreciated cooperation', can be dramatic.

- *Always speak respectfully about other ego states when talking with any state.*

  Ego states respond to praise or criticism in the same way people do. This makes intuitive sense since our experience of people is our experience of their executive ego states. It is often the case that when an ego state is speaking in therapy, other ego states are listening, especially when the conversation is related to them. Therefore, it is important to always speak respectfully about other ego states, even if they are causing havoc within the family of states.

Think about speaking to a person negatively about another person while they are listening. You would not expect to later get positive cooperation from the person who had been denigrated. This applies with ego states, and it can be an easy trap for beginning ego state therapists. It is easy to hear one state complaining about another and enter into the conversation against the state that has been causing havoc. This is not helpful for a positive resolution. Here is an example.

A person who is exhibiting obsessive compulsive behavior will often have an ego state that feels a need to check locks and water spigots before going to bed or before leaving the home. This 'Checker' state may compulsively check and recheck, taking much time and energy, and other states may become extremely angry with this state. While hypnotized, they may complain, show exasperation, even desperation about this 'Checker' state. The state that checks is doing so for a reason. It feels it has to check to protect the client in some way. It often will feel alienated in the family of states, but it feels it must do its job, sometimes fearing that if it doesn't the person will die. It feels what it does is important. If the 'Checker' state hears the therapist talking against it with other states it will harden its position and may not even choose to cooperate and talk. The chance of negotiation and inclusion is lost.

It is OK to listen to one state complaining about another state, but it is not therapeutic to become involved in the complaint. If a state says, "'Checker' is ruining everything. I can't even hold a job, because I can't get to work on time. I feel like giving up." A good response is, "I can see how that would be very hard for you. That must be extremely frustrating. I'm sure 'Checker' is doing what he has been doing for a reason. I'm going to be really interested in hearing about that reason. It would be good if we can find a way for all the states to help each other."

States will often disbelieve at first that a resolution can be found, "He will never listen to you. All he ever wants to do is cause trouble." A good response is, "Sometimes we can be pleasantly surprised. Is it alright with you if I speak directly with 'Checker' to see what we can work out?"

It is the role of the therapist to stay above the fray. States may, at first, seem like they will never accept a new function, or a new vision of another state. It is amazing how quickly this seeming intransigence can dissipate with respectful and creative negotiation.

- *Promote an internal dialogue, getting stronger states to help weaker ones.*
  The internal dialogue of the family of states is a fascinating feature of the psyche. Groups of states tend to work together, and communicate very little with other states, or other groups of states. Some of the underlying states may not even know other states exist. Some states have never communicated together. It is common for a state to view certain states as allies, and dislike other states. When a person says, "I wish I wouldn't do that. I don't like that part of me", one state is saying it does not like another state. When a person says, "When I get in front of a group something takes over and I can tell jokes and I get really energized", one state is saying that it likes and respects another state. When a person says, "When I get in front of a group something takes over and I can't speak. It is like I freeze", one state is observing another state, and is not able to understand what is happening.

A goal of Ego State Therapy is to promote positive internal dialog, and mutual respect of all states. When a person has states in conflict, it is at the very least, unsettling. When states communicate well and work well together, the client can feel integrated and confident.

50

It may be that the goal of therapy for some clients has nothing to do with resolving trauma from an earlier age. The goal of therapy may be to enhance internal dialogue and cooperation. The goal may be to achieve a happy working relationship among the family of states. States that have never communicated can be introduced, and, following negotiation, can work together for the benefit of the client.

It is interesting that states that have been introduced and that learn to communicate with each other continue this communication. Years later the client can be hypnotized and these states will report continued communication. A client reporting limited memories from a time in childhood may benefit from a childhood state being introduced to a surface state. Memories will continue to become available to the surface state as they continue to communicate.

Suppose a client has difficulty speaking in front of a group. When standing facing a group the client freezes up and words cannot be found to serve the client. The state that has become executive cannot deal with the group. It feels overwhelmed and incapable. The same client may have another state that can communicate in a relaxed fashion, a state that enjoys communicating.

These states can be introduced using hypnosis and Ego State Therapy. The state that freezes in front of groups can get help from the communicative state. The following is an example of how states may be encouraged to communicate, and continue to communicate after the session. Three states are involved in this process. They call themselves, 'Nervous', 'Talkative', and 'Librarian'. The client is hypnotized.

Therapist: Picture yourself now standing at the front of a room full of people. You can see their faces and you know they expect you to speak. Exactly how are you feeling?

Client: (In a low voice) My throat does not feel like working. My whole body feels flushed. I don't think I can talk. I feel really stupid.

Therapist: Thank you for talking with me, part that is feeling stressed in front of the group. What can I call you, as you stand there in front of the group?

Client: 'Nervous'.

Therapist: Thank you, 'Nervous'. Is it OK with you if I find another part that can help you there in front of the group?

Here, there is a choice of finding another part that can help, or going to the origin of the nervous energy. Either strategy can be effective. Resolving the original trauma is preferred, as discussed in section 3.1. Getting help from a different part without attending to the original trauma is quicker, easier, and effective.

Client: Sure.

Therapist: I would like to talk with a part that enjoys communicating. That is relaxed in communicating and likes to relate what you know. Just say, "I'm here", when you are ready to talk.

Client: (Silence)

Therapist: I would like to talk with a part that may just enjoy talking with a friend on the couch, a part that has really enjoyed being heard. Just say, "I'm here", when you are ready to talk.

Client: Yes, I'm here.

Therapist: Thank you for talking with me. What can I call you?

Client: (In a clear voice) You can call me 'Talkative'.

Therapist: Thank you, 'Talkative'. Tell me about yourself. When do you like to talk?

Client: I love to talk with my friends, about anything.

Therapist: That's great, 'Talkative'. Did you hear what 'Nervous' was saying about not being able to talk to people?

Client: I heard.

Therapist: It sounds like you have a natural talent for sharing what you know. Would you be willing to help communicate to groups? It would be very helpful.

Client: I don't usually talk to groups.

Therapist: I understand, but you are a very good and clear communicator. I can tell that by the way you talk with me. If I can help get you the information you would need to share, would you like to help?

Client: Yes, as long as I know what to say, I'll say it.

Therapist: I really appreciate that, 'Talkative'. That will be very helpful. Thanks for talking with me, and I will want to talk with you some more later. Is it all right with you if I talk with another state now?

Client: Yes.

Therapist: Now, I want to talk with a state that has the information to relay to the group. I want to talk with that knowledgeable part with thoughts or information to share with the group. Just say, "I'm here", when you are ready to talk.

Client: I'm here.

Therapist: Thank you for talking with me. What can I call you?

Client: I'm the Librarian.

Therapist: So, can I call you, 'Librarian'?

Client: Yes.

Therapist: Have you been listening to me talk with 'Nervous' and 'Talkative'?

Client: I've been listening.

Therapist: Do you know 'Nervous' and 'Talkative'?

Client: I know 'Nervous', but I don't know 'Talkative' very well. I knew she was there.

Therapist: What do you think about 'Talkative' taking a greater role in talking in front of groups?

Client: 'Nervous' sure doesn't like to do it. I get really frustrated trying to give her information. She just freezes up and won't say anything.

Therapist: So it would be all right with you if you could give 'Talkative' the information and she could share it with the groups?

Client: If she is willing to do that, I'm sure she would do a better job than 'Nervous'.

Therapist: Can you speak with 'Talkative' right now and see if you can work out a deal to do that, and then check with 'Nervous' to see if it is OK with her?

Client: I can try.

Therapist: Good. Go ahead and talk internally, and tell me when you are finished.

Client: (pause) It's OK with both of them. 'Nervous' was glad to get rid of the job.

Therapist: That's great, 'Librarian'. You will need to maintain more communication with 'Talkative' now, and I don't think you will feel as frustrated in sharing your information. Are you happy to do that?

Client: Yes, I can do that.

Therapist: Thanks again, 'Librarian'. I would like to talk with 'Talkative' now. Are you there, 'Talkative'?

Client: (loud and clear) I'm here.

Therapist: Is that arrangement all right with you? Are you willing to communicate more with 'Librarian' to get information when you talk to groups?

Client: Yeah, she said she will be happy to give me all the information I need. That was all I was worried about. I did not want to be there with nothing to say.

Therapist: Good. Now, when there is a group to be talked to, this is your role, to talk, and 'Librarian' will help with the information.

Client: I can do that.

Therapist: Thanks again, 'Talkative'. Now I want to talk with 'Nervous'. Just say, "I'm here" when you are ready.

Client: (quietly) I'm here.

Therapist: 'Librarian' said you are happy with the new arrangement. Are you willing to give up the role of talking in front of groups?

Client: I did not want it in the first place. If 'Talkative' will do it, she can do it.

Therapist: That's great. I want to thank you 'Nervous' for being helpful, and I want to thank 'Librarian' for agreeing to communicate more with 'Talkative' so 'Talkative' can talk to groups, and I want to thank 'Talkative' for agreeing to do that. Is there anything left undone in this process? Any part can answer.

Client: (no response)

The client is brought out of hypnosis.

Therapist: Now, picture yourself standing at the front of a room full of people. You can see their faces and you know they expect you to speak. Exactly how are you feeling?

Client: (Client smiles) I feel relaxed. I think I can do this.

- *Encourage states to trade or change functions, when helpful.*
  The above is one example of a state taking on the function of another state. Sometimes, as in the above example, states are happy to give up a function. At other times more negotiation is required.

  It is often helpful to find a new role for a state that is asked to give up a function when they are reluctant to do so. For example, a state that has expressed anger inappropriately may be asked to allow an assertive state to express feelings more appropriately. The anger state may be assured that it is still a very important state, and that if the person is ever in real danger the aggressive anger state will be needed. In this instance it is good to have a third state designated as the decision maker, deciding when the assertive state is needed, and when the anger state is required. States that can express much anger are not usually good at knowing when to become executive.

  A woman once came to me who clenched her jaw almost every night during sleep. She had tried hypnosis and other aids, but her jaw was often very sore, and her teeth were being ground. Her dentist had told her she would have to wear a mouthpiece at night, and she was concerned about being able to sleep.

  Using hypnosis and Ego State Therapy, I talked with the state that clenched the jaw during sleep and with another state that called itself 'Hedonist', quite a fun loving, and laid back state. The clenching state agreed to allow 'Hedonist' to have control of the jaw during sleep, in a trade for the hands. By communicating with each of the two states, I was able to gain assurance from 'Hedonist' that she would keep control of the jaw during the night, allowing it to remain relaxed. The tense state agreed to allow 'Hedonist' to have the jaw during sleep, in exchange for the hands. A general question was asked, if any other state objected to this arrangement. None did. The woman reported a complete and continued cessation of clenching her jaw during sleep.

- *Map the ego states, and keep track of which ones can communicate with each other, and what the roles of each are. You can later call on ego states you know for help.*
  It is important to take good notes on each state you talk with during a session. Often you will be able to call on a state from your notes, when needed, and at the end of the session you can refer to your notes to thank each state you have worked with, and remind them of how they have agreed to help. Ego state mapping can be beneficial on its own, as a device that allows clients to gain better personal knowledge and a greater ability to use their strengths (see section 3.3.1). Some therapists become known for ego state mapping and see many clients who want to become more personally aware, and more fully functioning.

  Learning states and being able to call on them has many benefits, including benefits in areas such as public speaking, parenting, sports psychology, studying for and taking tests, and social enjoyment.

2.2.3 The Dichotomous Technique for Accessing Ego States

One of the easiest ways to access separate ego states in hypnosis is with the *Dichotomous Technique*. It is a simple technique that uses a prior recognition of separate states by the therapist to bring those states to the executive, individually during hypnosis. It can be presented in eight steps. These steps will be presented, and then each step will be explained.

1. Interview the client and discover at least two of the client's mood states.

2. Introduce ego state theory, explaining how we are composed of separate mood states.
3. Hypnotize the client, and asked to speak to 'only the part that (for example) feels in control at work'.
4. Notice the automatic switching of the states.
5. After speaking to each state, ask what you can call it in order to refer to it in the future.
6. Thank the state for talking with you and ask its permission to speak to the next state.
7. Continue and speak with the next state in the same fashion.
8. After switching the client between states a few times other states may be talked with.

Explanation:

1. *Interview the client and discover at least two of the client's mood states.*

   Prior to hypnosis, discuss with the client at least two different states, for example for a particular person, a state experienced when feeling out of control with children, and a state experienced when feeling in control at work. These should be specific to the client. Information should be gathered relating to these states, such as where the client experienced them, with whom, the feelings experienced, the sensory perceptions; information that will enable you to "assist the client into the experience of the state while under hypnosis".

2. *Introduce ego state theory, explaining how we are composed of separate mood states.*

   Describe to the client how we normally change states and how it is important to be able to work with these states individually. Make sure the client understands that ego states are something that is normal and that we all are composed of these separate states.

3. *Hypnotize the client, and asked to speak to 'only the part that (for example) feels in control at work'.*

   Here you use the information gathered in step one to help the client into the state. It may be helpful to build the scene so the client can more easily slip into the ego state that you wish to speak with. For example, you may use the same adjectives

57

describing work that the client used. If you can incorporate different sensory perceptions, that can be helpful. Mention where the light comes in the room, the feel of the desk, the emotional feelings associated with that state. You will have gathered this information prior to hypnosis.

4. *Notice the automatic switching of the states.*
   Often a mind or cognitive state jumps in when the client is first learning to distinguish the states. When this happens reflect this to the client, "That seems like another part of you is talking now. Right now I really want to speak with the part that feels in control at work." Alternatively, you can talk with the state that has 'jumped in' and see what it has a need to express.

5. *After speaking to each state, ask what you can call it in order to refer to it in the future.*
   States sometimes have difficulty coming up with a name. You can offer suggestions given your knowledge of its function, as defined by the client. For example, if a state relates its role as 'saying what the client wants to say at any given time', you may ask it if it would like to be known as, 'Assertiveness'.

6. *Thank the state for talking with you and ask its permission to speak to the next state.*
   "I appreciate your talking with me, and I wonder if it is alright with you now for me to speak directly with that part of you that sometimes feels out of control with the children".

7. *Continue with the next state.*
   "Sometimes you are at home in your kitchen and the children are not listening to you. You are trying to cook and to get their attention, and they are pretending not to hear you. I would like to speak directly with that part of you that feels out of control. Just say, 'I'm here' when you are ready to speak." Here, again, you will be using the detailed information that you made notes on when talking with the client before hypnosis.

8. *After switching the client between states a few times other states may be talked with.*
   "Tell me exactly how you are feeling right now" is a statement that often results in a state expressing itself that has a need to

speak. You can also ask to speak with 'a state that has something to do with (or that knows about) the presenting problem'. For example, "When you came you said you have been having trouble with your anger. I would really like to talk with that part of you right now that can sometimes get really angry; that part that can get really loud and have high emotions. Just say, 'I'm here', when you are ready to speak."

2.2.4   The Resistance Deepening Technique

This technique is a hypnotic deepening technique that is presented here because it makes up part of the *Resistance Bridge Technique*, a technique for accessing ego states that need resolution. The Resistance Bridge Technique is presented in section 2.2.5.

Resistance is often viewed as something that should be avoided or sidestepped during the induction in order for hypnosis to begin. Induction techniques have been designed to avoid resistance, and a belief exists that the client who cannot achieve a clinical hypnotic state cannot do so due to resistance. Another way to view resistance is as an asset to the client and hypnotherapist, providing a focused path to a deeper state. The *Resistance Deepening Technique* (Emmerson, 2000) uses the resistance of the client to hypnosis as an induction focus. While all hypnotic inductions use focus, the Resistance Deepening Technique takes what the client cannot keep from focusing upon (resistance), and at the proper time, uses that as the primary focus. This is a deepening technique used in the final stages of induction, rather than a complete induction technique. The hypnotherapist may combine it with most inductions.

At the final stage of induction the client is asked, "I would like for you to tell me exactly what you are experiencing right now." The therapist listens for resistance in the response, such as, "My neck feels a bit tense", or "I'm a bit nervous about losing control." When resistance is heard, the therapist leads the client to focus directly on the subject of the response. An attempt is made to have the client increase the level of the reported experience. This facilitates a more narrowed focus, and a deeper hypnotic state. A more complete example of this technique is illustrated in the following section.

2.2.5   The Resistance Bridge Technique

Finding the origin of the client's presenting problem is imperative for the discharge of unwanted symptoms. Discovering and processing the unresolved trauma that is associated with a current pathology is a central feature of a number of therapeutic orientations, including psychoanalysis (Freud, 1901), Gestalt (Perls, 1969), and Ego State (Watkins and Watkins, 1997). When a trauma associated with pathology is resolved, the pathology becomes inert. The *Resistance Bridge Technique* is a hypnotic technique that assists the client in moving directly from the later stages of induction to the origin of the presenting concern; so unresolved issues may be addressed. It combines two techniques, the *Resistance Deepening Technique* (Emmerson, 2000), and the *Affect Bridge* (Watkins, 1971). The Resistance Deepening Technique uses the client's resistance to hypnosis as a focus to achieve a medium to deep hypnotic state, and the Affect Bridge assists clients in moving from the unwanted symptom to the origin of the symptom. This discussion outlines the Resistance Bridge Technique and gives examples of its use. Ego state strategies are presented, each contingent upon three general types of responses clients make during the later stage of induction to the statement, "I would like you to tell me exactly what you are experiencing right now."

Three major tasks hypnotherapists contend with are inducing a hypnotic state, deepening that state, and using the hypnotic state to locate the origin of the presented concern. Clients normally hold a belief concerning why the presenting problem exists. During the course of therapy what the client had thought to be the cause of the problem is often found not to be the major cause. It is more useful to allow the cause of a concern to be revealed during therapy than to use valuable therapy time discussing intellectualized speculations (the client's, or the therapist's) that are most often inaccurate.

The Resistance Bridge Technique is a tool that allows the hypnotherapist to facilitate a hypnotic state, deepen the hypnotic state, and locate the origin of the presenting concern, all within a single procedure. It is a seamless combination of two techniques, the Resistance Deepening Technique (Emmerson, 2000), and the Affect Bridge (Watkins, 1971).

The Resistance Deepening Technique is an induction technique that helps facilitate a medium to deep hypnotic state with practically every client, including those who are highly resistant. The Affect Bridge is a way to use the anxiety being experienced by the client to bridge to the original (normally childhood) trauma that fosters that anxiety.

After using the initial induction technique preferred by the hypnotherapist and client, the hypnotherapist ask the client a question roughly in this form; "I would like you to tell me exactly what you are experiencing right now?" The purpose of this question is to locate resistance. Common answers are usually of the following three types:

1. Really relaxed.
2. My right shoulder feels really tight (this type response can be of any physiological un-ease).
3. Pretty good, but I'm having some difficulty letting go (this relates to a resistance more psychologically based.

A therapist can respond to (1.) a relaxed response, (2.) a physiological response and to (3.) a psychological response in the following ways:

1. *The 'relaxed' response*
    Question: "I would like you to tell me exactly what you are experiencing right now?"

    Response: When the client responds indicating no resistance (Relaxed Response) the hypnotherapist should continue to look for resistance with questions like, "That's good. I wonder if you are aware of any reluctance to really completely letting go?" If the client is unaware of any reluctance to let go (rather rare) a good question is, "What part of your body would you say to this point is the least relaxed?" The hypnotherapist is searching for the aspect of the client that is the barrier between where he or she is and a very deep hypnotic state. Once a physiological resistance response or psychological resistance response is made then therapy will continue accordingly (see below). It is rare that resistance cannot be found, but in that case therapy would, of course, proceed without using the Resistance Bridge

Technique. Here is an example of working with a client who during the final stages of induction responds to the 'how are you feeling' question with:

Client: I'm feeling really relaxed.

Therapist: I wonder if you are aware of any reluctance to really completely letting go?

If the client is aware of any reluctance to letting go follow response (3.) below.

Client: No, I'm actually very relaxed.

Therapist: What part of you body would you say to this point is the least relaxed?

Client: I'm pretty relaxed all over.

Therapist: That's great. I know you want to focus on "*Client*'s presented problem" and that even when we are very, very relaxed there is a part of the body that is not quite as relaxed as the rest. Survey your body right now and tell me what part of you body is the part that is not quite as relaxed.

By reminding the client of the presenting problem, stress associated with that problem may be noticed by the client.

Client: I guess my stomach has some tension in it.

This is a physiological response, so therapy can continue with the example below. If the initial response to the 'how are you feeling' question was physiological then therapy could continue as follows:

2. *The physiological resistant response*
   Question: "I would like you to tell me exactly what you are experiencing right now?"

   Response: When the client responds with a physiological resistant response, the hypnotherapist should ask the client to focus directly on the physical sensation. "I would like you to have the courage to really go into that feeling of tightness in your right shoulder. Really experience it. Tell me exactly what it feels like." Other follow-up questions include, "On a scale of one to 100, how much are you experiencing it right now? Describe every aspect you can notice to me." Further statements include: "I would like you to see if you can have the courage to allow that right shoulder to be your real experience right now. See how completely you can go into that experience, just on its own." By using the aspect that the client can't keep from experiencing (the resistance) as the central focus, the client is able to let go of other concentrations and enter into a deeper hypnotic state. Here is an example:

Client: I'm feeling pretty good, but my stomach is tight and nervous.

Therapist: Tell me exactly what you are experiencing in your stomach.

Client: I feel like I could almost be sick. It is tight right in the middle and I can feel it all the way up into my shoulders.

Therapist: On a scale of 1 to 100, how much are you experiencing it right now?

Client: About 60.

Therapist: See if you can go inside it and turn it up to a 70. Really experience it more fully.

No response:

Therapist: What are you experiencing now?

Client: It is 70 now. I am really feeling tight and nervous.

The client is now overtly demonstrating affect and is ready for the affect bridge part of the procedure. If the client is not outwardly showing affect continue to encourage a stronger experience by increasing the number. Repeat the adjectives the client uses to help maintain focus. Speak with the same emotion the client uses.

Therapist: Stay in that feeling, feeling tight and nervous, feeling your stomach as you do with the sensation going all the way into your arms, how old do you feel right now?

63

Client: About 5 or 6.

Therapist: I would like you to go to when you had this tight and nervous feeling in your stomach for the first time, when you were 5 or 6. Allow yourself to hang onto that feeling, and you are 5 or 6 having it. Are you inside or outside a building?

Client: I'm inside.

Therapist: Are you alone or with someone else?

Client: There is someone else there.

Therapist: Describe exactly what is happening.

The client is at the origin of the problem. The trauma can now be resolved (see Chapter 3).

(c) *The psychological resistant response*
Question: "I would like you to tell me exactly what you are experiencing right now?"

Response: When the client responds with a psychologically resistant response, the hypnotherapist should ask to speak directly with the part that is having difficulty letting go. For example, if the client says, "There is part of me that is having difficulty letting go of control", a good response is, "I really appreciate that part, because it is there to protect you, and I would like to speak directly with that part right now, that part that wants to hang on to control." Here is an example:

Client: There is part of me that is having difficulty letting go of control.

Therapist: That is an important part of you and it is there to protect you. I would like to talk directly with that part that wants to keep control. When that part is ready to speak directly with me, just say, "I'm ready."

Client: I'm ready.

Therapist: Thank you for talking with me. What can I call this part that I am talking with that helps keep control?

Client: What do you mean?

Therapist: If I want to talk with this part again later, I need to know how to call on you. What can I call you?

Client: You can call me 'Careful'.

Therapist: Tell me what your role is, 'Careful'.

Client: I keep control.

Therapist: That is important, and I am sure you are very helpful. Tell me about your need right now to help.

Client: I'm afraid of what might happen if I don't keep control.

Therapist: That must be very tiring, having to maintain that control constantly. It would be really nice to be able to have a rest when it is safe. Right now, while I am here, you can stay just alert enough to have the control you like, and I will let you have a bit of a rest. We both want to help. What do you think about taking a well-deserved rest, while still being available if needed?

Client: I still need to be able to keep an eye on things.

Therapist: That's perfect. You keep an eye on things while at the same time having a rest, and I will do what I can to help. You know I am here to help.

Client: Yes, as long as I can keep an eye on things.

Here, the resistance in the induction was the ego state, 'Careful', doing its job of protecting the client from being exposed to fragile and emotional feelings. This ego state is talked with in a respectful and appreciative manner, and a negotiation brings about an agreement for 'Careful' to take a rest. The respectful manner that 'Careful' is addressed allows this ego state to trust the hypnotherapist and want to cooperate in the therapy. At no time is 'Careful' discounted, and at no time is the power of 'Careful' questioned. This would result in more resistance. When resistance is fought, it strengthens. By the therapist being an ally, 'Careful' is willing to take a rest and trust that the therapist will be helpful.

Therapist: Great. Thank you for talking with me 'Careful', and for helping and I hope you can have a good rest. I know you deserve it. Now that 'Careful' is able to really relax and take a good, deep rest, I would like to talk with the part that 'Careful' was protecting. There is an uneasiness or fear there. I would like to talk directly with that part now. I want to be helpful. When you are ready to speak just say I am here.

Client: *(begins to cry)* I'm afraid.

Therapist: I understand and I will not let anything hurt you. Thank you for talking with me. What can I call you?

Client: 'Afraid'.

Therapist: How old do you feel, 'Afraid'?

Client: I'm five.

Therapist: Tell me how you feel.

Client: There are too many people, and my mother has gone.

Therapist: Where are you?

Client: *(crying)* It's my first day of school. I want to go home.

The client has gone to the origin of the problem. The trauma of being at school for the first day has stayed with the client, and that traumatized ego state returns when there is a crowded room that is associated with feelings of insecurity. The client experiences the exact feelings of the first day at school, even though the adult client cognitively recognizes there is nothing to fear in the crowded rooms of today. In order to be free of the return of these traumatized feelings, it is important for the five-year-old ego state, 'Afraid', to become empowered and feel safe. Once 'Afraid' feels safe and empowered then crowded rooms will no longer bring out a traumatized state, since the client is not carrying that trauma. The ego state still exists, but it is no long traumatized.

HOW CAN 'AFRAID' BE HELPED?

Ego states rarely, if ever, disappear (Emmerson, 1999). While it may seem appropriate for a state to leave, this is probably not possible, and usually not preferred. An ego state is an integrated neural pathway of mood and thought and, while it is impossible to prove, it is most probably permanent. If a state believes you want to remove it, it will hide and become non-cooperative. Some therapists working with ego states report having asked ego states to leave and them doing so, although a more probable explanation is that they hide, since they can be accessed at a later time.

Even states that are causing discomfort are a part of us and while they may not be removed, they can change in function to become a positive and integrated part of our ego system. States that have been traumatized can be empowered. States that have poor or negative communication with other states can learn new roles and better ways to communicate and fit into the ego system. States that cause negative psychological or physical symptoms can learn new ways to use their energy.

'Afraid' is a traumatized state that needs to become empowered and feel supported. In order to assist a state to change it is important to talk directly with that state. There is little benefit in talking with a cognitive state about an emotional state, if change is desired. Following from the above example we have already established communication with the state at the origin of the problem, severe anxiety during the first day of school. Empowerment and the release of fear are accomplished with the state facing the fear and having the courage of expression. When the state discovers it cannot be hurt by facing the fear, the fear is removed. Support is received by asking another, nurturing state to provide the support the needy state requires. It is most important to find a state that 'wants' to help in this process. Finding a state that 'merely agrees' to try and help will not result in a permanent solution, since that state will most usually tire of helping and later stop. Here is an example of this process:

Client: *(crying)* It's my first day of school. I want to go home.

Therapist: Tell me exactly what is happening. I am with you and I am not going to let anything happen to you.

Client: *(crying)* My mother left. I did not want her to go and I don't know anyone.

Therapist: Staying right where you are, I want you to know that this is only a memory. It is a memory you carry with you and we have power over it. What do you need right now with your mother gone?

67

Client: I need my mother back.

Therapist: It is not fair that she left you there alone with those people, is it?

Client: No. She should not have left me.

Therapist: I would like for you to see your mother standing right in front of you right now, and I want you to tell her what you feel.

This ability to express pent-up feelings helps empower the client who feels abandoned and weak.

Client: I'm afraid to tell her.

Therapist: I'll tell her first then you can tell her. What can I call her?

Client: Mum.

Therapist: Mum, you should not have left when you did!! You should have stayed longer!! Now you tell her. Tell her what you feel.

Client: I want you here. You had no right to leave. You should have stayed.

Therapist: That's good. What is she doing? What is she saying?

Client: She says she did not want to leave. She thought she had to.

Therapist: Say what you want to say to her?

Client: You do not have to leave Mum. I want you.

Therapist: What did she say?

Client: She says she is sorry.

Therapist: How do you feel about your mum now?

Client: I love her.

Therapist: Can you ask her for a hug?

(Pause)

Therapist: What is happening now?

Client: She hugged me and told me she loves me.

Therapist: That's good. Can you hug her back?

Client: *(smiling)* I am.

Therapist: What do you feel about the students and teacher who are there right now?

Client: I don't know them.

Therapist: Would you like them to be your friends?

Client: Yes.

Therapist: Tell them how you feel, like you told your mother how you feel.

Client: *(speaking to the students)* I'm scared, and I need a friend.

Therapist: What is happening?

Client: A little girl named Emma says she would like to be my friend.

Therapist: That's good. Would you like someone to stay with you there who you can trust?

Client: Yes.

Therapist: Thank you, 'Afraid', for talking with me. I want to talk with you some more later, but right now I want to talk with another part of you. I want to talk with an older, nurturing, part that likes helping children. I want to talk with a part that would like to help 'Afraid' on her first day at school. Just say I'm here when you are ready to speak.

Client: *(in a clear voice)* OK. I'm here.

Therapist: Thanks for talking with me. What can I call you?

Client: You can call me 'Helper'.

Therapist: 'Helper' have you heard what has been happening with 'Afraid'?

Client: Yes.

Therapist: Would you like to help her feel better at her first day at school?

Here is where it is important that the state wants to help, rather than is merely willing to help. Otherwise, the intervention will not be permanent.

Client: Yes.

Therapist: That's great. I want you to go to 'Afraid' now and tell her you will stay with her. You can give her a hug if it seems right.

(Pause)

Therapist: What is happening now?

Client: I'm with 'Afraid'. I have my arm around her.

Therapist: 'Helper', are you willing to be with 'Afraid' any time she needs you?

Client: Yes, I would like that.

Therapist: Thank you, 'Helper'. I would like to talk directly with 'Afraid' now. Just say I'm here when you are ready.

Client: Yes, I'm here.

Therapist: What is happening now, 'Afraid'? Is 'Helper' there with you?

Client: Yes, she has her arm around me.

Therapist: From now on she will be with you anytime you want her. How does that feel?

Client: (relaxed and smiling) It feels good.

Therapist: How do you feel now?

Client: I feel good. I'm not afraid anymore.

Therapist: Since you don't feel afraid, would you like a new name?

Client: Yes.

Therapist: What would you like to be called now?

Client: I want to be called 'Loved'.

Therapist: OK. From now on when I want to talk with you I will call you 'Loved'. 'Loved', you were brave and told your mother how you feel, and have found she is sorry for leaving. You have found a friend, Emma. And you have 'Helper' to be with you anytime you want. Is there anything else you need?

Client: No.

Therapist: 'Loved' I want to thank you for talking with me and for your honesty and bravery, and 'Helper' I want to thank you for your help, and continued help. And 'Careful' I also want to thank you for the work you do and for helping me by taking a well-deserved rest.

It is now time to bring the client out of hypnosis. The client will no longer be carrying these unprocessed feelings. They will no longer manifest themselves during times when the client is in a crowded room with unknown people. She will be able to remain relaxed and will be able to respond appropriately to the situation at hand. The ego state that continued to hold fear and trauma and a feeling of abandonment from being with unknown people now feels empowered and nurtured.

The trauma that precipitated these unwanted reactions was not brought about by any parental neglect. Indeed, if the parent had acted exactly the same with another child, or with this child on another day, no trauma may have been sustained. Yet, an ego state was traumatized and was able to benefit from processing and empowerment.

This was an example of the Resistance Bridge Technique, and of empowering a traumatized state. There are many different ego state techniques for processing trauma, and several will be presented in the following sections. Other than for processing trauma, Ego State Therapy is beneficial for improving state-to-state communication (e.g., "I don't know why I act like that. I don't like myself like that", or "sometimes I feel like I have to have him in my life, and sometimes I know I never want to see him again"). It is also good for helping clients to better understand their states to get the best use of each. Dr. John Watkins and Helen Watkins (1997, 1990, 1982, 1981) and other therapists (Emmerson and Farmer, 1996; Gainer, 1993; Frederick and McNeal, 1990; Newey, 1986) have provided many illustrative works to assist in the use of Ego State Therapy.

For a transcript example of the Resistance Bridge Technique see section 4.5.1.

2.2.6 *Accessing States that are Reluctant to Speak*

One of the most difficult aspects of Ego State Therapy is accessing reluctant states. It may sometimes not be possible to gain access to the state that really needs treatment. There are some techniques that help make it possible to communicate with even the most reluctant state. A client will sometimes have a state that the existence of is denied. For example, if a client wants to quit smoking and has had difficulty quitting, there is a state that wants to, or likes to, smoke. That client might respond to the statement, "I would like to talk with a part of you that sometimes wants a cigarette" with the statement, "There is no part of me that wants to smoke." If no part (ego state) of the client ever wanted a cigarette, then the client would not smoke.

Another example is the client who gets so nervous when attempting to talk in front of a group that words are difficult to find. When this nervous state comes to the executive the client will demonstrate emotional tension. If the client is speaking in a relaxed and confident manner, then the nervous ego state that needs attention is not yet executive.

The following are some causes that ego states may be reluctant to speak, may find it difficult to speak, or may be unable to speak:

1. The level of hypnosis may not be deep enough.
2. The ego state that is currently executive does not want to give up the executive.
3. The desired state may believe the therapist does not like it.
4. The desired state may believe the therapist wants to get rid of it.
5. The desired state may not have communication with the currently executive state.
6. The desired state may not be listening.
7. The desired state may not know it can speak.
8. The desired state may not be able to speak.
9. Another state may attempt to block the therapist from speaking to the desired state in order to protect it from pain.

Explanation:

1. *The level of hypnosis may not be deep enough.*
    One of the most common reasons ego states do not come to the executive and speak is related to the level of hypnotic trance. Without hypnosis, or in a light state of hypnosis, only surface states (see section 1.1.2) are accessible. Some states require a deeper state of hypnosis to become executive. For most ego state work it is not necessary to for the client to experience a deep level of hypnosis, but research has indicated that practically every client can achieve a deep level of hypnosis with a good indirect induction (Fricton & Roth, 1985). There are several good hypnotic deepening techniques that may be used when there is a concern that the hypnotic state may not be deep enough. One such technique (the Resistance Deepening Technique) is discussed in section 2.2.4.

2. *The ego state that is currently executive does not want to give up the executive.*
    A client may have a state that is nervous about giving up the executive. Such a state may at first deny that any other states exist, and may find it safe to hang onto the executive. This executive state may have fear about what might be found in underlying states. When this occurs I say something like, "I want to say to this protecting state that I appreciate the good work you do protecting this person, and I know that work must be tiring. I'm sure it would be nice to be able to take a rest at a time when you know it is safe, at a time when someone else can help look after the more fragile parts. You know I am here to help and you can help too, now by taking a much-deserved rest while I talk with some other parts. It is all right for you to be ready, while you rest, to come back and protect this person if you are needed. Now is a real opportunity for this person to gain some relief and you can help with this just by resting. So now, with you listening from the background, I would like to speak directly with *desired state*. Just say 'I'm here' when you are ready to speak."

3. *The desired state may believe the therapist does not like it.*
    It is important to always speak respectfully to and about all states. If you speak negatively about a state to another state it may not be willing to talk with you when you ask. It may not come to the executive. Even if you always speak respectfully

about it, it may believe, given its role, that you will not like it. When calling such a state to the executive it can be helpful to explain how important the state is, and how you need its help. "I would like to speak with the state that sometimes gets very angry. I know you are very powerful, and I know you do your best to protect this person. You have a very important role. I know you do what you do to help this person, and I need your help now so we can help this person together. Just say 'I'm here' when you are ready to talk."

4. *The desired state may believe the therapist wants to get rid of it.*
    A number of times I have had an ego state express to me a fear that I might try to get rid of it. This fear is sometimes given as an explanation why it did not want to speak with me. Occasionally a different state will, when I am calling the desired state to the executive, report "he is afraid you will make him go away". It is not unusual for a second state to respond for the desired state in such a manner. When this happens I continue talking with the intermediary state until the desired state gets tired of using the intermediary and begins speaking directly. When the state has fear that I will try to make it go away, I respond with something such as, "I don't want you to go away. You are very important, and I need you to help this person. I need your help. You have power and energy that can be very helpful. We don't want to lose that. Will you help me? Just say 'I'm here' when you are ready."

5. *The desired state may not have communication with the currently executive state.*
    Remember the metaphor of the classroom of students, as the family of states within a person. Just like in a classroom of students, groups of states often know each other well. If you are speaking with an ego state that is easily familiar with the desired state it is normally quite easy to transfer communication from that state to the other. If, though, you are speaking with a state that has little or no communication with the desired state, calling out the desired state is not as easy. I normally say something such as, "I want to speak with the state that has something to do with the procrastination. You may be in the background, so you may need to listen carefully. If there is another state that knows the state that has something to do with the procrastination please help get that state's attention. I want to talk with a state that

knows about the procrastination, or a state that knows about that state now. Just say 'I'm here' when you are ready to speak."

6.   *The desired state may not be listening.*
     There are different reasons a state may not be listening. It may be well removed from the states you have been speaking with, as in number 5 above. It may not know how to speak, as in number 7 below. It may believe it cannot understand the language being spoken. Occasionally, when a client was raised speaking a different language, early states may believe they cannot communicate. They will be able to communicate either with another state acting as an interpreter, or they often find, when they try, they are able to communicate in the current language. Usually after another state acts as interpreter for a few sentences the desired states begins speaking directly, and understandably.

7.   *The desired state may not know it can speak.*
     Some states report being infants, at an age prior to the development of speech. Other states may become aware of the infant state wanting to speak, and may interpret for the infant state. Often after interpretation progresses the state that reports being an infant will respond to a suggestion that although it could not speak as an infant, it will be able to speak now. It is possible to work with states using a different state as an interpreter, but it is much easier to be able to speak directly with states that are important to the treatment of the individual.

     Finger signals (autonomic finger signals) may be used in the initial contact with a state, prior to asking it to continue communicating with speech. "I am interested in the state that knows something about the development of the obsessive compulsive behavior. If this state can hear me please raise the index finger on the right hand." If the index finger raises, "That's good, I can see you can hear me. I would like to speak with you directly. Just say, 'I'm here' when you are ready to speak."

8.   *The desired state may not be able to speak.*
     If all efforts at getting a state to speak directly fail, continue to use a state that can communicate with the desired state as an interpreter, or continue to use the autonomic finger signals.

These are not the preferred ways of communicating with a state that is needed for treatment, but they may, at times, be the best available. After using this method of communication during a session, a suggestion may be given at the end of the session that the state that was not able to speak may learn to speak prior to the next session, and that other helpful states may be instrumental in bringing about this learning.

9. *Another state may attempt to block the therapist from speaking to the desired state in order to protect it from pain.*
    It is common for fragile states to have other states that protect them. These protector states are useful and needed, but they can block access to states that need help. The affect bridge and the resistance bridge technique (section 2.2.5) are two methods of bypassing these protector states. Addressing protector states in the method illustrated in number 2 above (the ego state that is currently executive does not want to give up the executive) is another useful technique to provide access to states that are blocked by others. Section 3.1.4 contains a discussion about working with protector states.

Chapter 3

Using Ego States in Therapy

This chapter defines some of the uses of Ego State Therapy and outlines how therapists can apply the therapy. Examples are given to help clarify therapeutic techniques.

Ego State Therapy allows the therapist and the client near complete access to the different parts of the personality. This greatly increases the ease and speed of positive change. In order to help a client who is having difficulty with anger, it is much more powerful to speak directly with the state that expresses anger. Speaking with an intellectual ego state about anger, or about a time when the person was angry is akin to speaking to one student in a class about the behavior of another student. Just as it would be much more productive to speak with the student who is having trouble in order to change the behavior, it is much more productive to speak directly with the ego state that is associated with unwanted symptoms in order to change those symptoms.

Some therapists have learned to access the ego state that needs help without being aware of Ego State Therapy. The angry ego state will often become executive by asking the client to explain in detail what happens when anger is expressed inappropriately, or by asking the client to describe an occurrence in detail and affect. At this time good therapeutic change can take place.

If an ego state carries trauma, pain, anger, frustration, or hurt this toxic baggage can prevent the individual from being able to live fully and functionally. This baggage can be manifested in the form of physical symptoms, disease, headaches, or other hysteric symptoms. It can be manifested psychologically in the form of neuroses, and the fear of facing this unprocessed baggage can prevent the person from having access to some loving and useful states. Allowing those fragile, loving states to become executive can be too scary.

3.1   Processing Trauma

Everything we do is connected to a cause. When we consistently react in a way that is inappropriate to the situation, it is because an unprocessed trauma is present within the ego family of states. There is no "statute of limitation" on processing trauma. Trauma may be processed years after the original occurrence, and while what happened may always be appreciated as negative, it does not have to continue to interfere with current living. It may be the case, "once cut, always scarred". A scar is a reminder of a cut that has healed. It is not the case, "once cut, never healed". An unresolved trauma is a cut that has not healed. Traumas can be found, processed and healed. The knowledge of occurrence will rightly continue, but the disruptions of an unhealed, unprocessed trauma can be replaced with an ability to react physically and emotionally in a manner appropriate to the situation at hand.

3.1.1   Abreactions

An abreaction is a negative emotional or physical response in therapy that is related to an earlier trauma. Abreactions may occur while working through a trauma. In ego state theory, the mere act of experiencing an abreaction is not considered therapeutic, but the act of resolving the trauma, which often entails abreactions, is therapeutic.

Examples of abreactions include a client suddenly beginning to cry deeply, a client showing immense fear, or a client moving physically in a manner not associated with the current situation. A client's hand might start jerking, or a client might appear to move back into the chair, into a seemingly safer position. Another example would be if a client were to scream, or yell out, normally in apparent fear.

It is important for the therapist to be able to remain helpful and attentive to the client during times of emotional release if ego state work is to be conducted. With ego state work the client can rather quickly move from the trauma of an abreaction to a feeling of being expressed, empowered, and calm. It is gratifying to be a participant in this change and to understand that the toxic trauma that once fueled the abreaction, and any associated neurotic reactions or panic attacks, has been replaced with feelings of peace and empowerment. This change appears to be permanent. In order for this change to take place the therapist must be able to stay with the client during the abreaction and find out what is needed and supply those needs. This is often done by encouraging expression to any internal abuser, by encouraging the client to express needs and to act upon them (such as loudly telling the abuser to leave), and by getting help for the client from stronger ego states to gain a feeling of peace and calm (see section 3.1.4).

Abreactions are relatively common when doing ego state work. They can be thought of as markers or flags indicating where work needs to be done so the client can feel settled and so the trauma does not continue to lie underneath, waiting to be expressed in a problematic manner. Abreactions often occur when a trauma is revisited so that empowerment over fear can result. If the trauma were not processed, merely revisiting the traumatic event and the related experience of an abreaction would leave the troubled ego state unresolved, and would leave the client feeling closer to the original negative experience. It is therefore very important to resolve a trauma when it is revisited. When a trauma is resolved no further abreactions associated with that trauma will occur. Neurotic reactions, panic attacks, and PTSD symptoms can be thought of as abreactions outside of therapy, since they are reactions related to unresolved trauma, and the resolution of the associated trauma will result in their cessation.

3.1.2   Neurotic Reactions

A situational neurosis is a repeated inappropriate response to a particular type of life situation. A neurotic reaction of this type is directly tied to a lack of resolution being held by an ego state that becomes executive when cued by some situational cue. When cued, this ego state will re-experience the same feelings of the original occurrence. For example, a client of mine became extremely anxious when attempting to speak in front of groups. It did not matter how much he prepared, he would become fearful, shake, and feel like no matter how he tried he could not be good enough.

We discovered, using ego state techniques, that once as a child when he was working with his father in a field, a trauma was created and not resolved. His father was having a bad day and my client could not please him. His father continued to yell at him no matter what he did. The boy became very frightened, physically shook, and did not think he could talk to anyone about it without getting into more trouble. The state was unresolved and throughout life when my client felt he would be judged for a verbal performance this unresolved boy ego state would come to the executive with the same feelings he had in the field. By following the steps for trauma resolution set out in following sections my client was able to enjoy talking to groups in a confident fashion. The previously unresolved state, after reaching resolution, was no longer cued to come to the executive when he spoke to groups.

3.1.3 Finding the Trauma

Finding the trauma that is associated with a particular neurotic reaction is a real strength of Ego State Therapy. A direct link may be made between the unwanted symptom and the originating unresolved trauma that continues to cause the unwanted symptom. This link can often be made in a single session, and resolution can begin immediately. Components of ego state techniques to find a trauma are varied. The Resistance Bridge Technique (section 2.2.5) in this book details a technique for finding a trauma associated with a traumatic reaction. The Resistance Bridge Technique is highly recommended for locating this type of trauma.

It is also possible to locate and resolve trauma without knowledge of how that trauma may be impacting upon the life of the client. Unresolved trauma can result in psychological and physical negative symptom etiology, it can be a cause of panic attacks, and it can result in more general unsettled feelings. Resolving trauma allows the client to operate in a more fully functioning manner, with better psychological and physical health. The following is a technique for finding trauma using guided imagery. Once a trauma is located, steps for resolution presented in the next section may be used.

FINDING A TRAUMA BY WORKING WITH IMAGERY

Ask the (hypnotized) client to imagine walking through a deep forest along a clear path. Continue with something like, "As you walk down the path you notice the sound of your footsteps and you become aware of the surface on which you are walking. You become aware of the material that makes up the surface and the exact noise it makes as you walk on it. You may notice the amount of light coming through the trees, and the feel of the air on your skin. The air has a certain temperature and I am not sure if it is still or moving against your skin."

Continue building a sensually detailed imagery walk and then begin asking questions, such as, "There is something there in the trees you have not noticed before. You can focus on it now, and tell me what you want to tell me about it." After bringing the client verbally into the imagery experience begin asking for a sense of what is good and bad along the trail. "I want you to situate yourself on the trail so you can see some distance in different directions; where you can see clearly and not so clearly various things in the distance. There may be something either close to you or in the distance that you have a good feeling about. What is that?" Allow a short explanation about what is good on the trail. This 'good' questioning is only to prepare the client for the next question.

After the client has had a short opportunity to describe something that was perceived as 'good' on the trail say something like, "There may be something either close or in the distance that is frightening to you, or that you have a bad feeling about. I am not sure if you can see it from where you are standing right now. It may even be over the hill or behind something, or even in a cave. I would like for you to tell me about that now." The client may just have a feeling that there may be something bad in the distance.

A goal of this process is to find a fear. Fears we carry are related to unprocessed traumas. Continue directing the client to what is the most frightening. If it is in a cave ask the client to have the courage to enter the cave. Explain that you will be with them. Bring the client as close as possible to the fantasized fear, then (if necessary to get stronger affect) see if the client can increase the fearful feelings on a scale of 1 to 100 to a higher number. Whenever the client shows significant affect (emotion) go through the line of questioning, "How old do you feel? Go to when you were (that age) feeling like this for the first time. Are you inside or outside? Are you alone or with someone else? Tell me exactly what is happening there as a (that age) year-old." Of course you will vary and pace these questions according to the responses you receive from the client.

FINDING A TRAUMA WORKING WITH DREAMS

The imagery trip is a good technique to find unprocessed traumas. Dream processing is another way to accomplish the same thing. Most dreams offer a symbolic release of anxiety. When participants in research are deprived of REM (rapid eye movement, when dreaming occurs) they become more and more anxious. Dreams are associated with anxieties that have not been resolved. It can be suggested to ego states that dreamtime can be used to play, work, or be mischievous if a state cannot resolve the amount of time spent on these activities with other states. Clients who can remember their dreams will then report more of the nominated activity in the dreams.

Anxieties may be located and resolved using a process similar to the one with imagery above. A fearful part may exhibit that fear in a symbolic form in a dream. When the client reports the fearful dream, the therapist should work to increase the feeling of affect so that it will be able to lead to the unresolved cause of the 'bad dream' with the use of a bridging technique.

3.1.4 Tools for Processing Trauma

Finding trauma is only the first step in resolving unwanted symptoms. Some theoreticians believe that merely finding trauma and becoming aware of how it has affected the life of the client is therapeutic. They believe that "insight fosters resolution". Other theoreticians believe that "revisiting trauma re-traumatizes. Ego state theory holds that it is not enough to merely gain insight, that revisiting a trauma without resolution may leave the client feeling re-traumatized, but that it is important to revisit a trauma in order to gain resolution. Trauma resolution is a goal of Ego State Therapy. There are three important elements in processing trauma. The three essential elements for processing trauma are:

1. *The traumatized ego state must be executive for trauma to be processed.*
    Probably the biggest waste and mistake in therapy is spending time working with a state that does not need help, talking about a state that does. Because of this, many clients spend weeks, months or years in therapy with work taking place in the wrong place. Find the state that has the trauma and make sure it is the state that gains resolution. The Resistance Bridge Technique (section 2.2.5) discusses how to locate and gain access to a traumatized state.

2. *The client must rise above fear and express true feelings to any person associated with the trauma.*
    When trauma is present it is important for the client to be able to feel expressed; able to say anything that fear kept the client from saying previously. It is important that the client is able to demand of any antagonist what is needed by the client (e.g., that the antagonist leave). Often it is very useful for the therapist to demand (in a loud voice) of the antagonist what the client wants, prior to the client own expression. For example the therapist may say to the antagonist who the client has described, "You had no right to do what you did", then to the client, "OK, now you tell him what you want to!" It is imperative that the traumatized state express for itself, but it may not be able to express before the therapist leads the way. When the traumatized state becomes stronger than the fear, the fear loses its power.

3. *It is important that any remaining needs of the traumatized ego state be met, normally by other stronger ego states.*
    After the client has, while speaking from the traumatized ego state, been able to rise above fear and express to the aggressor there is often a residual feeling of exposure, or loneliness. Good questions to help define what is needed are, "Tell me exactly how you feel now", or "What do you need right now?" When the previously traumatized ego state is able to define what is needed the therapist can call for an ego state that would like to provide that need to the needy state. For example, "I would like to talk with a mature, nurturing part that likes to help young children. When you are ready to speak, just say, I'm here." The states should be introduced, and a process of negotiation should leave both

feeling positive about an ongoing relationship of meeting each other's needs.

CONFRONTING THE PROVOCATEUR

Trauma is often maintained because the traumatized ego state of the client feels powerless in relation to what I will call the *antagonist*. The antagonist may range from a loving parent who took the child to kindergarten on the first day, to the sadistic abuser. The antagonist may also be something other than a person, like a dog or a storm.

Common to the antagonist is the feeling of powerlessness and lack of resolution the client felt at the time toward this person, or thing. The client continues to live with a feeling of powerlessness and incompleteness until processing occurs.

It is important that the processing occurs with the client's internal antagonist. That is, if the child was eight years old, the processing needs to occur with the antagonist that surfaced when the client was eight. It is OK for the client to literally and physically go back and talk with the person today who was the antagonist of years ago, but this will not resolve the trauma. The trauma is held in the ego state that was traumatized, and it is this ego state that must gain resolution.

I do not encourage, or discourage, clients to confront the real people of today who were the antagonists of the past. For instance, if a client wants to bring legal charges, I see that as a decision outside of therapy. It does not resolve the trauma held by the traumatized state. It may allow the adult to feel an appropriate course of action has been taken. It may also result in pain and frustration. If the antagonist is a perpetrator, and is believed to be a current danger to the client or to someone else, then it is appropriate for innocent people to be protected.

It is imperative that the client be in the traumatized ego state when working to process the trauma. This state will exhibit much affect and it is necessary for the therapist to be able to encourage the client to stay in that state. Some therapists feel uncomfortable when the client is uncomfortable, but to assist the client in releasing trauma, the traumatized state must be executive.

Once the fearful state is able to express to the antagonist what it really feels, the fear disappears. This dramatic change was, at first, difficult for me to understand. It is actually quite simple. Fear of the antagonist is held, until the antagonist is no longer feared, then it is released. When clients have the courage to face the antagonist and say whatever they want, then they have overcome their fear, and it no longer exists. When clients rise above fear, they become the more powerful, and they naturally do not fear what is weaker than they are.

How do we help traumatized ego states face their antagonists? They are often reluctant to say anything, because of the fear. I tell them, "I am going to be with you", and, "I am not going to let anything hurt you". A good question to ask is, "What do you want to say?" If the client is too frightened to express, I will often speak to the antagonist first, after asking the client, "Would you like me to tell them first?" Then I will say, in a loud and commanding voice, something like, "You had not right to do that. You should not have done that". Then I will say to the client, "Now you tell them what you want to tell them".

I continue to encourage the client to say what is felt, and I encourage the client to do with the antagonist what is desired (usually "yell at them to go away"). And if I think it will be helpful, I continue to tell the antagonist to do the same things the client is telling the antagonist to do ("You don't belong here. Go away. You can't stay here. NOW LEAVE!)." I continue to ask the client, "What is happening now?" It is almost always the case that when the client asks the antagonist to go away that the antagonist goes away. The client has become the more powerful and the fear disappears. It is important to continue working with the client until the desired outcome is achieved.

THE MISUNDERSTOOD ANTAGONIST

The antagonistr may be a parent who is trying to act in a loving manner. Consider a parent who takes the child to kindergarten the first day. This can be a traumatic experience for a child. A parent scolding a child can result it that child-internalizing trauma. Sometimes a parent does not know how to show love and communicate well. That parent may be too harsh, but is still a parent who loves the child. The most common traumatic experience

85

I have found that clients return to is that of being left in a room alone, calling out, and the parent not responding.

There is no way a child can be raised without the experience of trauma. We have all experienced trauma. It is only when the trauma goes unprocessed that it may return as unwanted symptoms. Trauma that results from misunderstood antagonists requires a varied treatment.

It is still important for clients to be able to express themselves to the antagonist, even the misunderstood antagonist. It is still important for clients to be able to use other of their ego states to make sure needs are met on an ongoing basis. What is also important in trauma resulting from a misunderstood antagonistr is that it is beneficial for clients to gain an understanding of the disposition of the antagonist.

After clients have been able to express themselves to the misunderstood antagonists it is helpful for them to take on the antagonist's identity. The antagonist within the client is an introject (see section 1.2), and while an introject is not a true ego state the client can assume the identity of the introject and experience feelings such that the true person may have had at the time.

It is interesting that, upon assuming the identity of the introject, the client is able to express thoughts and feelings beyond those understood by the client's troubled child ego state. For example, the child ego state may see the parent as mean and unloving, and may say that the parent "does not love me". Upon assuming the identity of the introject the tears stop, the affect changes, and the client often expresses, as the introject, frustration at the child, love for the child, and a concern over the problems of the introject. When asked, "Why are you yelling at Susan (the child)" the introject may say, "I had a really bad morning. I don't want to yell, but that is the way my parents talked to me." Below is an example of dealing with a misunderstood antagonist.

Sue is a client who was becoming very upset at work when her boss pressured her to work faster. She knew she was over reacting. She had experienced these strong feelings throughout her life, especially when she felt pressured. She felt very nervous and upset, often when she felt people pressured her to work faster. An affect bridge (Watkins, 1971) was used to connect the current negative feelings to the original occurrence (see section 2.2.5).

During hypnosis, Sue was encouraged to relate a time at work when she feel upset about being pressured. She was asked to describe the feelings in detail. She spoke about a time when her boss had rushed her to get a form to her, making Sue very upset.

Therapist: Feeling upset by your boss right now, tell me exactly how you feel.

Client: I can't do anything right. I can't do anything fast enough. I know she does not like me.

Therapist: On a scale of 1 to 100 how strongly do you experience those feelings right now?

Client: Pretty strong. About 70.

Therapist: You can't do anything right. You are too slow. You know you are not liked. Can you get that number up to 80?

Client: *(crying)* I'm there.

The client is encouraged to increase the feeling until clear affect is observed. Then the next step can proceed.

Therapist: How old do you feel right now, feeling you can't do anything right?

Client: I don't know. Not very old, about seven, I guess.

Therapist: Right now, you can't do anything right. You are too slow. You know you are not liked. I want you to go to when you were about seven having those feelings for the first time. Are you inside or outside a building?

Client: *(crying)* Outside.

Therapist: Are you alone or with someone else?

Client: *(crying, very upset)* I'm with someone else.

Therapist: Tell me what is happening.

Client: My dad is yelling at me for not getting out of the way!

Therapist: What can I call you there feeling the way you do at seven?

Client: *(still crying)* You can call me Susan.

Susan and seven are written on case notes and circled.

Therapist: Susan, what do you want your dad to know?

Client: *(still crying)* I don't know. I am moving as fast as I can.

Therapist: Tell him! Tell him what you need him to know.

Client: He'll just yell at me more.

Therapist: This is your chance to tell him. I am here with you. I won't let anything happen. Tell him directly that you are doing the best you can.

Client: *(crying)* I am doing the best I can. I'm just little.

Therapist: What is he doing?

Client: He's just looking at me.

Therapist: What do you feel about him?

Client: I hate him.

Therapist: Tell him how you feel about him. Tell him everything you feel.

Client: I hate you! You should not yell at me! I can't do what you want.

Therapist: And now what is he doing?

Client: He is still just looking at me.

Therapist: Right now I want you to become your father who is there looking at his little girl. I want you to be him. When you are the father, say 'I'm ready'.

Only ask the client to assume identity of the introject of another person when you feel they will gain from deeper understanding by doing so. I do not ask clients to assume the identity of an introject, such as a perpetrator, who appears to only have bad intentions.

Client: *(stern and cold)* I'm ready.

Therapist: What can I call you, father?

Client: You can call me 'Dad'.

Therapist: Dad, did you hear what Susan just said to you, that she hates you?

Client: I heard.

Therapist: How does that make you feel?

Client: I don't want her to hate me. She just gets in front of me and I can't get to the door.

Therapist: What do feel about Susan?

Client: I love her.

Therapist: Why is it hard to show her that?

Client: Nothing ever goes right for me.

Therapist: This isn't going right, is it?

Client: No.

Therapist: Would you like to tell Susan that you love her?

Client: Yes.

Therapist: Go ahead and tell her now. Tell her out loud so I can hear you.

Client: I love you Susan. You are all I have.

Therapist: Can you tell her that you are sorry for yelling at her?

Client: I'm sorry I yelled, Susan. I did not want to scare you.

Therapist: Thanks Dad. I may want to talk with you some more, but right now I want to talk with Susan again. Are you there, Susan?

Client: I'm here.

Therapist: Did you hear what your dad said?

Client: I heard.

Therapist: He really does love you, and he is sorry about yelling at you. What do you think of that?

Client: I don't know why he has to yell at me.

Therapist: He really does love you, Susan. He is not perfect.

Client: I know. He makes me really upset.

Therapist: Tell him.

Client: You make me really upset!

Therapist: Does he make you upset because you love him and you don't want him upset with you?

Client: Yes.

Therapist: Tell him.

Client: I love you Dad. I wish you wouldn't yell at me.

Therapist: Can you give him a hug?

Client: No.

Therapist: That's OK, why not?

Client: I'm a little afraid.

Therapist: Would it be OK if he gave you a hug?

Client: Yes.

Therapist: I would like to say directly to Dad that Susan would like a hug. If you can do this, go ahead. (Pause) What is happening now, Susan?

Client: He is hugging me.

Therapist: How does that feel?

Client: It feels good.

Therapist: What do you want to say to your dad now?

Client: I love you Dad.

Therapist: What do you need now?

Client: *(smiling)* Nothing.

Therapist: Dad, are you there. Please answer me directly.

Client: Yes, I'm here.

Therapist: How does the hug feel to you?

Client: Great!

Therapist: Are you willing to continue showing your love to Susan in an appropriate way? She needs to know you love her.

Client: Yes.

Therapist: Susan, your dad will always be there for you inside and show you his love from now on.

Client: *(still smiling)* I feel really good right now.

Therapist: I want to thank you Susan for having the bravery to talk with me, and for having the bravery to tell your dad your feelings and what you need. I also want to thank you for being able to help your dad show his love to you. And I want to thank you, Dad, for your help, and for your continued help in letting Susan know that you really do love her.

Therapist: Sue, I want you to picture yourself at work. Your boss is pressuring you to get the form to her, right now. You are at work. How do you feel?

Client: Smiling. I'm not upset. I want to get the form to her, but I feel OK.

The client was taken to a time when she would normally feel upset to check on the effectiveness of the procedure. The unresolved ego state of Sue (Susan) that felt she could not please was no longer lingering in her with negative feelings. That part was finally able to feel resolved, so Sue was able to respond in a manner appropriate to the situation. Once a resolution such as this is achieved, it is seems to be permanent.

GAINING HELP FROM OTHER EGO STATES
One of the most powerful tools in ego state work is being able to call upon other ego states to help a needy state. Help may be sought to provide nurturing, to provide task related skills, to provide assertiveness that can release pent-up feelings, or for a number of other needs. An internal negotiation can result in a new

internal cooperation that is beneficial to every ego state involved, and thereby, to the person. It is most appropriate for this internal assistance to be sought only after the resolution of any related trauma. For example, a client will normally have a nurturing state that enjoys nurturing children, and enjoys gaining the benefit of feeling useful and appreciated by a child. This nurturing state may be used internally to nurture a needy child state, with both states enjoying benefits from the interaction. The child state gets needed attention, support, and love, and the nurturing state gets to feel appreciated and useful. Still, a nurturing ego state will not be able to help a particular child state relax and feel comfortable if the antagonist is still internally threatening the child state. The child state must first be able to completely and accurately express feelings to the antagonist and the antagonist must either be driven away or must become understood as harmless. After the toxic fear of the antagonist has been eliminated, it is often the case that the abused child state will continue to feel needy. This is when help may be called for from other internal ego states, such as a nurturing state. It is now possible to answer the following:

- *When should internal help be sought from other ego states?*
  It is useful and appropriate to seek internal help for an ego state from another ego state when the needy state has resolved trauma issues and when an internal need exists.

- *How do we know an internal need exists?*
  We know an internal need exists by hearing that need from the client. We may hear this as a response from a question such as, "How do you feel now?" We may hear that a need exists from non-elicited verbal communication, such as, "I'm still lonely". Or, we may hear that need exists from the body language of the client, such as speaking in a nervous voice, or body posture that reveals a non-comfortable, non-relaxed state. It is always good to ask a state that has been needy about how it feels after an intervention, and, whenever possible, make sure the state feels comfortable and relaxed before the session is brought to a close.

- *How can we ask for internal help from another ego state?*
  Before seeking help from another ego state it is important that (a) the client is hypnotized, (b) the client has already been switching between states (see section 2.2.3, The Dichotomous

Technique), and (c) that a need for help exists (see paragraph above). A general request for help for an ego state that has expressed a need may be asked, such as, "I would like to talk with a part that would like to help." This question calls for a state that is not only willing to help, but that wants to help.

An even better way to call for help is to phrase the call for help in such a way that it is clear, specifically, what kind of help is needed. To nurture a frightened child state, it is important to find a state that enjoys nurturing. If a strong state that does not enjoy nurturing volunteers to help, that state may be warmly thanked for offering, and told that you really need to talk with a state that would enjoy helping to nurture. "I need to speak with a state that cares about children and would really enjoy staying with this child state." It is important that the helping state wants to help and would enjoy helping, rather than merely agrees to help. A state that wants to help will continue to help far into the future. A state that sees helping as a difficulty often will stop helping in the short-term.

When calling on a state that you would like to speak with, it is important to give a clear understanding of how that state is to respond. Without this, the state may not become overtly verbal. After saying, "I would like to talk with a part that..." the state becomes aware that you want to talk with it. The next step is to inform the state how to respond when it is ready to speak. You may do this by saying something like, "When you are ready to speak, just say I'm here." After the state responds with, "I'm here" a conversation may ensue.

- *Do not give up looking for a helpful state.*
  Most often (when you call for help from another ego state, specify the exact help you need, and ask for it to respond with "I'm here" when it is ready to speak) after a short pause a state that wants to help will respond. Occasionally, no response will be forthcoming. When there is no response, I normally say, "Tell me exactly what is happening now." If the client responds that no state is coming forward, it can be that a state that would like to help did not hear you. All states are not listening at all times. Or it can be that no state exists that would like to take on the function you are offering.

It is best to first check to see if a state exists that would like to take on the function. A good follow-up question is, "There may be a state back in the background who can hear me now that would like to help. I want all states that might want to help to hear me now. If there is a state, even deep in the background that would like to help (you may be specific asking for the type of help) just raise the right index finger, the pointing finger on the right hand. If there is a state that would like to help that state can raise the right index finger now please" (autonomic finger signal). If the index finger rises, then you may begin speaking with this state. "I see, the index finger did raise. I want to say thank you to that state that raised the index finger. Please say, 'I'm here' so we can talk directly."

If a state does not come forward who wants to help, a state with a different function may want to take on a new role and help. It is good to ask for a state that has not had this role in the past, but would like to be more useful and would like to take on the desired role now.

• *Accept help only from states that want to help.*
It is not enough to get a state that is willing to help, since a state that does not really want to participate in a role will not do it very long. A state that wants to help will normally continue helping.

A state that feels exposed and needy for love may be helped by a state that likes to nurture. A state that is swimming and afraid of drowning may be helped by a state that is a good swimmer. A state that is cold may be helped by a warm state that can bring a large blanket. A state that is lonely may be helped by a state that would like a friend. It is important to find the need, and whatever that need is, find a state that wants to satisfy that need.

WORKING WITH PROTECTOR STATES
Protector states were formed to keep the person from experiencing pain. They often protect the fragile ego states by keeping people away from these fragile states. Protector states also may keep the client from being able to experience deeper feelings of love and joy, since they keep fragile, tender states from coming to the executive. It is the fragile, tender states that are sensitive enough to

94

experience these feelings of love and joy, but these are the same states that can most easily experience pain. It is for this reason that protector states are useful. It is important to address protector states in ego state work for two reasons.

1. Protector states often attempt to block the therapist from reaching the fragile states that have been traumatized, and that need resolution.
2. Protector states need to learn to work with the family of states to allow fragile states into the executive when it is safe so feelings of love and joy may be experienced. These same protector states need to be available to protect these fragile states when it is not safe, when the fragile states might feel overexposed.

WHAT DISTINGUISHES A STATE AS A PROTECTOR STATE?

Sometimes when you asked the state for a name it will give the name, 'Protector', and this state will almost always be a protector state. Often other names are given, such as 'Anger', 'Fear', or 'Checker'. Of course, some clients give states personal names such as 'Fred', 'Mark', or 'June'. More than anything else, it is the role of the state that defines it as a protector state.

We need protector states. They are good for us, and they are necessary. They, like most other states, began as coping mechanisms at a time when the client needed them. They sometimes adopt roles that are problematic. The checking state of a person with obsessive-compulsive disorder is a protector state. By compulsively checking this state is attempting to protect the person from some internal or external pain. A withdrawn state is a protector state that attempts to protect the person from a threatening situation by withdrawal. The expression of anger can be a coping tool of a protector state.

When a state holds unresolved trauma protector states are needed to keep current situations from reactivating the pain, and to hold the pain away from current executive ego states. Protector states need to be educated about the importance of their roles, and about how they can best fulfill their role of protection. If an anger state becomes overt too often, it may be problematic for the person. An assertive state may learn to work with an anger state so reactions appropriate to the situation may occur (see transcript in Chapter 4).

How do we get past a protector state so we can work with a state holding a trauma? A client who has difficulty reaching a medium to deep state of hypnosis often is blocked by a protector state that makes a barrier between the therapist and the trauma. Using the Resistance Deepening Technique the therapist may asked the client to report, "Exactly what are you experiencing right now?" This is a way to hear from the protector state that is blocking the progress of the hypnosis. The following is a dialog with a protector state:

Therapist: Exactly what are you experiencing right now?

Client: I don't think this is going to work.

Therapist: Tell me exactly what is happening.

Client: I just can't seem to let go and get into it.

Therapist: I hear that part of you wants to let go and something is keeping that from happening. I would like to hear what is happening that is keeping you from being able to 'let go and get into it'.

Client: I start thinking this is just silly.

Therapist: It sounds like there is a part that does a good job of protecting you, keeping you away from what is deeper. I'm sure that part is important and has done a good job in the past. I want to talk directly with that important part that has been keeping you from going deeper by saying 'this is silly'. I just want to talk with the part of you that thinks this is silly. It will be the part that responds with 'yes' when I ask, 'do you think this is silly'? Part, do you think this is silly? Just allow that part to respond.

Client: Yes, it's silly.

Therapist: Thank you for talking with me, part. I know you are here to protect this person in some way. Can I call you 'Protector'?

Client: Yes.

Therapist: Protector, you must do a very good job of keeping this person and others from what is inside, and that is an important job. Right now, I want to help this person so what is inside can feel better. It must take a lot of energy and work always being vigilant, protecting the inside. I'm sure it would be nice to just be able to take a rest and help me help this person. Would you be willing to help me help this person by now taking a bit of a rest? That will give you a well-deserved rest and it will help me be helpful. You can still keep an eye open if you like so you can make sure everything is all right. Is it OK with you if this person is able to go deeper now?

Client: Yes.

This sequence of questioning may sound unusual, but it normally results in the person immediately being able to reach a deeper state. This type of permission to go further may be used at any time in Ego State Therapy, and can be useful in getting past protector states even when the client is already in a deep state of hypnosis.

It is common for protector states to keep other people away from fragile states. These protector states may be educated to allow fragile states into the executive when it is safe and keep them from the executive when it is not safe. Often a protector state will need help from another ego state to be able to do this, since the protector state may not be able to decide when it is safe. The following is an example of this type of ego state work. This example comes from a segment with the client hypnotized and Ego State Therapy in progress:

Therapist: What can I call this part I am speaking with right now?

Client: You can call me 'Careful'.

Therapist: Thank you for talking with me, 'Careful'. What is your role?

Client: I keep the little girl safe.

Therapist: That sounds like a very important role. I have spoken with 'Little Girl' and she can benefit from your protection. She is lucky to have you to keep her safe. She also needs love. I wonder if you would be willing to let her come out and get a hug or love when it is safe, but for you to be there to protect her and keep her from coming out when it is not safe.

Client: I'm afraid she might get hurt. She has been hurt a lot.

Therapist: I understand that. And you are right. She has been hurt and we don't want her to get hurt. But she also needs love. I wonder if you would be willing to work with another part that could help you decide when to let her out to experience good things, and when to keep her in to protect her.

Client: Maybe.

Therapist: Thank you, 'Careful', for talking with me, and I will want to talk with you some more, but right now I want to talk with another part. I want to talk with a part that is smart enough to decide when it is safe for 'Little Girl' to come out. I want to talk with a part that would like to work with 'Careful' so 'Little Girl' can get some love. Just say, "I'm here", when you are ready to talk.

Client: I'm here.

Therapist: Thank you, part, for talking with me. What can I call you?

Client: You can call me 'Inner Strength'.

Therapist: 'Inner Strength', did you hear me talking with, 'Careful'?

Client: I heard.

Therapist: Are you able and willing to decide when it is safe for 'Little Girl' to come out, so you can tell, 'Careful'?

Client: I can do that.

Therapist: Is that something you would like to do, because, unless you would like to do it, I would rather find another part?

Client: No, I would like to do that.

Therapist: That's great, 'Inner Strength'. Right now I would like you to talk directly with 'Careful' and I don't have hear what you are saying. See if you can work out the details of your making the decision about when it is safe for 'Little Girl' go come out and telling 'Careful' so she can do the important job of protecting 'Little Girl'. Just say, "We're done", when you are finished talking with 'Careful'.

(Pause)

Client: We're done.

Therapist: Were you able to work it out?

Client: Yes.

Therapist: That's great. I really appreciate you help, 'Inner Strength'. Now, I would like to talk with 'Careful' again. Just say, "I'm here", when you are ready to speak.

Client: Yeah, I'm here.

Therapist: 'Careful', what is the arrangement you have with 'Inner Strength'?

Client: She is going to call me when I need to protect 'Little Girl' and I am going to let 'Little Girl' come out when she says it's safe.

Therapist: That's great, 'Careful'. It sounds like you are going to be able to do you job even better. You will be able to protect 'Little Girl' and let her get love too.

Client: Yeah.

At this point both states are thanked for taking on their new roles and are again reminded of their new roles ("I want to thank both 'Careful' and 'Inner Strength' for..."), and the hypnotic session can move to the next task or can be ended.

3.1.5 When is Processing Complete?

Determining when trauma processing is complete is dependent on several things. A single incident of trauma may require only a single trauma resolution session. A single traumatic incident can have a profound influence on the life of a client, and it is possible for that negative influence to disappear completely after a single trauma resolution session. A client who has experienced a number of traumatic incidents may require a number of sessions, especially if different ego states were traumatized. The following procedure may be helpful.

First, get a clear definition from the client concerning the nature of the present negative feelings. When do they occur? How are they experienced? Get a detailed account of the client's physical, and emotional feelings.

Second, use the Resistance Bridge Technique or the Affect Bridge to locate the origin of the trauma within hypnosis. Process the trauma. Make sure the troubled ego state has been able to be completely expressed, and make sure the ego state has all needs met, by a greater understanding, with the help of a misunderstood antagonist, or with the help of one or more able ego states. It is important that the client, while in the state that was traumatized, feels complete resolution. This may take one or more sessions.

Third, hypnotically place the client in a current situation that would have previously brought about the negative feelings. See if the negative response has been extinguished. Sometimes a trauma is resolved, and it is not actually the trauma that was the causal agent for the negative feelings. This third procedure ensures that the proper trauma has been resolved. If a different trauma was resolved, good work has still been done, both by the client and by the therapist. You can ask clients to do a life survey to see if, or when, feelings of the type that were experienced in the trauma, were felt again during other times in life. You can ask them if they were felt recently. This allows both of you to know how the client was helped by the trauma resolution. When the client moves directly from the current feelings to the trauma using an affect bridge, it is almost always the case that the trauma resolution resolves the unwanted reactions.

If the client has a number of issues, several trauma resolutions may be required. If the client does not gain a feeling of complete resolution for a single issue, more than a single trauma resolution may be required. The client should consistently be heard to in making these determinations.

3.2   Improving Ego State Communication

Section 3.1 provided a discussion of one of the three functions of Ego State Therapy, to locate ego states harboring pain, trauma, anger, or frustration and facilitate release, comfort, and empowerment. This section provides a discussion of a second function of Ego State Therapy, to facilitate functional communication among ego states. The common phrase "he is at peace with himself" or "she is at peace with herself" refers to good ego state communication. A person can be internally settled when ego states respect each other and communicate in a productive fashion. Examples of comments people may make that signify non-functional ego state communication are, "I don't know what gets into me. I wish I wouldn't say those things. I don't mean them", "I hate that part of me that gets so upset", "Part of me wants to finish school, and part of me just wants to take off", "I love him, I hate him, I love him, I hate him", "I know I have to get this work done, but I get into a state where I just don't want to do anything."

One of the most powerful examples of a person with poor ego state communication is a person who might be diagnosed as having obsessive-compulsive disorder. This person may have a state that has a great need to repeatedly check locks, or to enact some other behavior in a compulsive manner. The state that acts compulsively may be hated by other states that just want to get on with life. This person will not experience a settled peace within until the states learn roles that can be respected by all states.

A common physiological response to poor ego state communication is headache, tension or migraine. Other physiological symptoms may also result from poor ego state communication, or from unresolved trauma (see section 3.1). Experiencing internal peace promotes better psychological and physiological health.

Our internal family of states is not unlike a large nuclear family group. Within a person may be a family of states that communicate and function well, or there may be states that feel alienated, or subgroups of states that operate in opposition to other states. It is important to remember that all states started for the benefit of the person. All states see their role as important. Sometimes states do not understand the role of other states, and sometimes states assume roles that may be detrimental to the person (see section 3.2.3).

Improving ego state communication involves gaining the confidence of each state. States may need to change their roles. States will need to learn to respect and cooperate with other states. This work can be frustrating, and it involves good negotiating skills, but it can facilitate internal peace.

3.2.1 Negotiating among Ego States

Ego state negotiation is when the therapist acts as a negotiator for the client's internal family of states in order to bring internal resources to needs. It is important to be able to negotiate among the ego states of a client. Ego states may need to learn to respect each other, exchange roles, help each other, and learn good communication skills.

1. *Ego states need to respect each other.*
    When an ego state does not respect another ego state the person does not respect an aspect of self. An ego state of a person may want very much to do well on an upcoming exam. Another ego state may very much want to go to a movie or spend time with a friend. The state that wants a good result on the exam may resent and dislike the more social state. This internal dissonance creates an unsettled feeling that moderates self-respect. Ego state negotiation may be used to help each state understand the value of the other, to learn to communicate with each other, and learn to share time in a manner that each can feel positive about.

2. *Ego states may need to change roles.*
    A client may feel very nervous when talking in front of a group and may feel unable to have good self-expression while in front of the group. The same person may very much enjoy talking to a friend while setting on a couch at home, and at that time may have the ability to be verbal and articulate. It is possible for the verbal and articulate ego state to take on the role of talking in front of groups. The ego state that had been nervous talking in front of groups may quite enjoy a different role. Negotiation can result in two or more states exchanging roles. Sometimes a state is quite happy to give up a role it does not enjoy without taking on a new role. Some ego states will need to have another role before they are willing to give up a role.

3. *Ego states may need to get help from other states.*
    Our family of states is complex and dynamic. Some states may feel weak and fragile, while others feel strong and assertive. We may have a state that enjoys nurturing, and another state

that needs nurturing. A fragile state in need of nurturing may feel great relief when a nurturing state meets that need, and the nurturing state will normally gain from the internal interaction as well. Ego state negotiation can make sure that these states each get what is needed.

4. *Ego states need good internal communication.*
    Ego states not communicating properly can be compared to members of a family not communicating properly. Misunderstandings can develop. States may take on roles for which they have little competence. The benefits of cooperation are not fully realized. Ego state negotiation can facilitate states that have never communicated with each other to begin, and continue, an internal dialog, and it can facilitate states to learn to work together in a positive way.

FACILITATING POSITIVE NEGOTIATION

The first step in facilitating positive negotiation among ego states is to gain the confidence of the states with which you will be working. Individuals who have poor internal ego state communication and poor respect between states will normally have states that feel alienated and non-appreciated. These states are often reluctant to speak, and sometimes report fearing that they will be asked to leave. It is important to give assurance that all states will be respected and that no state will be asked to leave. Never speak derogatorily about a state to another. If one state is complaining about another state, it is good to listen and show understanding, but do not make statements that could be heard as taking a position against a state. The following is an example (hypnotized client) of speaking to an ego state that is disapproving of another state:

> **Client:** I hate that part of me that always gives in to those people who put pressure on me.
>
> **Therapist:** That sounds frustrating, finding yourself committed to doing things you really don't want to do.

(An inappropriate response would be, "Yes, that is not a good thing to do." This response would tell the listening ego state that you are disapproving of it.)

Client: It is! I just wish I did not do it.

Therapist: I'm sure there is a reason you do it. I would like to learn about that reason. Is it all right with you if I talk directly with that part of you that sometimes gives in to people?

Client: Yes.

Therapist: Thank you. Right now I want to speak directly with that part that sometimes gives in to others. I know there is a reason you do this and I want to hear about it. Please just say "I'm here", just the part that sometimes gives in, so we can talk.

Speaking respectfully to (e.g., "Right now I want to speak directly with that part that sometimes gives in to others.") and about (e.g., "I'm sure there is a reason you do it. I would like to learn about that reason.") states helps the therapist gain access to states and helps the therapist engender a positive working relationship with states. Negotiation may proceed once the therapist has established this positive relationship. Ego state negotiation can be thought of as attempting to facilitate the best possible relationship for a group of people who stay in a single dark room. You may talk with each person and asked that person what he or she does, about other people who are known, and you can attempt to improve existing relationships and create new and positive relationships. These are goals of ego state negotiation. Patience, respect, and creativity are needed. The rewards can be profound.

3.2.2   Encouraging States into Alternate Roles

One of the most powerful aspects of Ego State Therapy is the rapid manner its techniques can result in ego states taking on new roles, and letting go of old ones. States may be asked to help other states internally, thus taking on the role of internal nurturer, or protector. Other ego states may be convinced to cease negative or harmful functions (see section 3.2.3), and take on positive functions.

The important aspect to remember when encouraging states into new roles is to make sure the state actually wants to take on the new role. If the state merely says it will try, then the change will likely be transitory. It is important to negotiate with the state to find a role that it believes it can do and that it wants to do. This process may require patience and creativity, and it may be facilitated by some states' willingness to trade roles or functions with other states.

3.2.3 *Working with Difficult and Malevolent Ego States*

One of the difficult aspects of ego state theory and therapy that new practitioners can find difficult to understand is that underlying states may dislike and even want to hurt other ego states. These difficult or malevolent states may be spoken with directly, and when they tell what they do, and why, it is easy to gain a broader appreciation of the complexity of the personality. The reasons for previously misunderstood statements and behaviors become more clear, both to the therapist and to the client.

Self-injurious behavior, obsessive checking, psychosomatic illness, suicidal ideation, and socially acting out in a manner that is often later regretted are just a few examples of the internal work of ego states that may be difficult or malevolent. Ego State Therapy brings light to the subconscious interactions that result in these types of behaviors. It provides techniques for working with these states directly so difficult and malevolent states may be brought back into the family of states as positive and productive members.

THE DEVELOPMENT OF DIFFICULT AND MALEVOLENT EGO STATES
Why would one of our ego states want to hurt us? Why would one of our parts act in ways that we would later deeply regret? Why would one of our parts play a role in making us physically ill, in giving a headache or a backache? It seems incomprehensible that we would be our own enemy without even knowing it. How could this personality structure develop?

A 32-year-old male client presented with the issue of binge eating. He had become overweight and he was concerned with his weight and health. The initial interview revealed that he ate in a healthy manner, with the exception of the bingeing. He did not suffer from the often-related problem of purging.

Hypnosis and ego state techniques (talking with different states, and calling for a state that knew about, or had something to do with the bingeing) located an ego state that claimed to have something to do with the bingeing. The state called itself 'Fishie', 'Fishie' was an example of a Creative Form Identity (CFI) (Emmerson, 1999). CFI's are ego states that express themselves symbolically through such forms as animals or body parts (e.g., an arm, or the chest). 'Fishie' reported being responsible for my client's bingeing. When asked "Why?" Fishie said it needed more room in which to "swim around", and this need for room resulted in bingeing. Further questioning revealed that Fishie felt a need for more room because this state was lonely and wanted to be able to swim around to look for a friend.

Fishie is an example of an ego state that was causing psychological and physiological problems. A lonely child ego state had represented itself as a fish in need of a friend. The under-developed logic of this state resulted in the belief that bingeing could increase the possibility of finding a friend. Ego state treatment involved negotiating with 'Fishie', and offering a friend to stop the bingeing. Fishie was happy to agree. All it needed was not to be lonely. The following statement was made, "I want to speak with a state that would like to be friends with 'Fishie'; a state that would enjoy staying with 'Fishie', playing and keeping him company." The bingeing stopped with Fishie's needs being met.

A 36-year-old female client presented with obsessive-compulsive disorder. One of her states called itself 'Checker'. Checker compulsively checked locks and water faucets or taps. It was possible to determine the internal dynamics of this client's family of states using Ego State Therapy. When my client was a small girl her father would become irate and yell violently. There was no physical violence associated with the psychological violence. My client had a state that was extremely distraught by the yelling, and had no state that had coping skills, so Checker was created.

The distraught state would call upon Checker, a trance-like state, so my client would not have to deal with the cognitive dissonance of a loved father yelling violently. The nervous, distraught state became Checker's internal friend, and Checker its friend. Checker was almost entirely mindless and was not capable of becoming executive without the distraught state calling it out. All surface states very much disliked Checker, because this state kept my client from being able to get to sleep at night, made her late for work or appointments, and caused her to feel generally out of control in life. Checker had come into being, like other ego states, to help my client cope with a difficult situation, and by continuing to do what it knew how to do, it brought psychological distress.

A self-mutilating state can begin in much the same way. Self-mutilation can be an escape from internal pain (by going into a trance state), it can be expressing anger one state feels toward another (or others), or it can be a combination of both. The ability to think clearly varies greatly among ego states. Some are wise and logical, and some states may be mechanical and initially unable to think. Occasionally an underlying state will express a desire to kill another state, or even all other states. This underlying state may believe it can kill the client without hurting itself. As we will learn below, these ego states have the potential to learn new skills, insights, and roles.

GAINING ACCESS TO DIFFICULT AND MALEVOLENT EGO STATES
Before negotiating with difficult or malevolent states to foster new insights, skills, and roles it is necessary to gain access to these states. It is often more difficult to gain access to these states than any other states. An ego state that has become disliked both internally, by other ego states, and externally, by other people, may expect little positive outcome from making itself available for communication. It is not unusual for these states to fear that a therapist will try to get rid of them. They often feel, also, that it is necessary for them to continue with the role they have. They often feel it is all they know how to do and that if they are stopped they will be useless, or the client may be placed in danger.

- *The first step in gaining access to a difficult or malevolent state is to hypnotize the client and begin talking with other ego states.*
  Do not attempt to talk with a difficult or malevolent state before the client has exhibited a good state of hypnosis and is easily switching between states. This is a good rule to follow when seeking to communicate with any underlying state.

- *Make general statements indicating your desire to work positively with all states and that you do not want to get rid of any state.*
  When you are ready to speak with a state it is likely that it is listening to what you say before you call it to the executive. By being clear that it is not your intention to get rid of any state, you will be more successful in being able to talk with a difficult state. The following is an example of this type of statement. "I want all states to know that every state is important and I do not want any state to leave. I need the help of every state, and I want to work with each state in order to help with the problem."

- *Ask to speak directly with the difficult or malevolent state.*
  If another state has already told you about the difficult state, it is good to thank that state for the information and ask if it is all right if you talk directly with the difficult state. States almost never refuse this request, and it helps them feel you are not 'taking sides'. They will be more cooperative with you later when you need their help. Then you can say something like, "I would like to now speak directly with the state that is causing the headaches. Just say 'I'm here' when you are ready to speak."

  If no state has told you of the existence of a difficult state you can make a general statement asking to speak with the state related to the concern: "I would like to speak with a state that either causes the self-cutting, or with a state that knows about that state. I know this must be a powerful state and I would really like to talk with it, or find out about it. Just say 'I'm here' when you are ready to speak."

  It is not unusual for a state that knows about the difficult or malevolent state to speak when the difficult state is not ready to speak. You can ask this knowledgeable state to translate between you and the difficult state. Normally, this translation last only a few sentences before the difficult state tires and begins speaking directly to you. This can be recognized by a chance in tone and wording, such as 'I do' rather then 'he does'.

NEGOTIATING A NEW ROLE FOR DIFFICULT AND MALEVOLENT STATES
As discussed in Chapter 1, I do not believe a state can be destroyed or removed. States will sometimes say they will leave, but these

states seem to be lying in wait, and can return to speak again if they are asked. Therefore, I believe when states agree to leave, the problem has merely been shelved, and not resolved. Since unresolved issues or states can cause a feeling of unrest, and can cause psychological or physical distress, I much prefer assisting states into positive roles, rather than attempting to remove them or ask them to leave. Assuring states that they will not be asked to leave, results in their being more prepared to talk and work positively.

States that cause problems for the client are usually disliked by other states, sometimes by all other states. This can cause the difficult state to feel isolated and misunderstood. This knowledge gives the ego state therapist additional leverage in facilitating a change in role, since it appears that states desire to be liked. They may, at first, deny this desire to be liked. The following are some steps in negotiating with difficult or malevolent states.

- *Gain the confidence of the state.*
  I like to express to the state the respect I have for some aspect it possesses. Here is an example: "I can tell you are a very powerful state. I really want to help this person and I need your help to be able to do that. I don't think I will be able to help this person without your help."

- *Appeal to the state by reminding it of its mission.*
  Ego states came about to help the person. By reminding the state why it is here, it often becomes more willing to fulfill its mission, and help the person: "I know you started to help this person, and I don't know if you realize now, but some of the things you are doing are actually hurting this person. I want us to be able to work together so we can both help this person."

- *Remind the state of its relationship to other states.*
  States liked to be liked and appreciated. Difficult and malevolent states are rarely appreciated. Often one of these states will claim it does not care what other states think about it. Don't believe it. I have never found a state that did not soften with the appreciation of other states: "It must not feel very good to be disliked you other states. Wouldn't it be nice to have a role where you could work with other states and where they would like and appreciate the things you do?" Common answers to this question include,

"I only know how to do one thing, and that is what I do."
(States can learn new roles even when they do not at first think
they can.) "They would never like me." (States are amazingly
quick to change their opinion of a state that takes on a positive
role.)

- *Help the state find a new role it can be good at.*
  By understanding what a state does you will be better able to
  find a positive role the state can fulfill. A state that is capable
  of making the person sick may also be capable of making the
  person feel better. A state that helps the person from experiencing pain by self-mutilating may be good at creating a
  trance. This state may be able to help the person rest by going
  into a trance in a safe place while listening to music.

- *Encourage new internal relationships once the state has taken on a
  positive role.*
  Ask other states what they feel about the new role. Encourage
  them to befriend the changed state. Ask the previously malevolent state how it feels being liked and appreciated by the
  other states. Encourage the states to help each other now that
  new roles have been developed.

- *Ask the state if it would like a new name.*
  Often states that take on new roles like to change their names.
  A state that called itself 'Mutilator' may want to call itself
  'Music Listener'. Sometimes a state that keep the same role
  but learned to apply it at appropriate times will want to keep
  the same name. 'Stubborn' may have learned to be stubborn
  when it is appropriate, and not at inappropriate times. 'Anger'
  may have learned to express itself overtly only at times of danger, and may express itself with the help of an assertive state
  at other times. These states, therefore, may want to keep the
  names of 'Stubborn' or 'Anger'.

It can be gratifying to work with difficult and malevolent states. It
takes patience and creativity, but the outcomes can result in the
disappearance of unwanted symptoms, and in the client feeling at
peace with self, possibly for the first time in memory.

3.2.4 When is Ego State Communication Good Enough?

Poor internal communication results in the client's feeling unsettled, in his having difficulty finalizing decisions, or in his failing to benefit from strengths. These are the markers that indicate that ego state communication is good enough. Unresolved trauma can also result in a client feeling unsettled. When the client is able to feel internally at peace, this is an indication that internal traumas have been resolved and ego states have respect for the roles each state has. Each ego state should respect the roles of the other states and a spirit of cooperation and understanding should be evident in the internal family of states. The following general question should be met with silence: "Are there any states that are uncomfortable with the role or function of any state? I would like to hear if any state is uncomfortable with any other ego state. Just say, 'I'm here' if you are not happy with the roles or functions of any state."

3.3 Gaining Personal Awareness of Ego States

Persons who do not know their ego states do not know themselves. We may know much about how we respond and to given situations. We may know what we expect of ourselves, but without knowledge of our personal ego state map and with knowledge of the feelings and traits of our individual states we cannot have a real understanding of self. It is important to remember that every person has a different ego state family structure, or ego state map. Each person's ego state structure developed according to that person's needs to cope with life circumstances.

In order to better illustrate how each of our ego state maps differs, and to better illustrate the value in understanding our ego state structure, I will discuss some of my own ego states. Before I learned my states I had a general understanding of how much I would allow myself to be exposed in a relationship, because I knew I could be hurt. I was somewhat conservative in allowing myself to be exposed, since I had learned what being hurt felt like. I was living blindly. Then I had an ego state mapping. I called two of the states I learned about, 'Fragile' and 'Infant'.

Both 'Fragile' and 'Infant' have a lot of fear. They have been hurt in the past and are afraid of being hurt again. They both also have much affect. Infant feels more than any other of my states that I know. While they both have fear and can be hurt, they are also both able to feel love in a powerful way. One of my greatest joys of living is when 'Fragile' or 'Infant' can experience love. These are states I very much appreciate having.

'Rationality' is an emotionally cold, mental state. It works quite well in thinking and weighing criteria. Feelings are held in the background when I am in my 'Rationality' state. That is to say, feeling states are not executive. Sometimes when 'Rationality' is executive, I do not experience feeling states as even existing. And sometimes a feeling state has so much need to be executive, I cannot stay in my 'Rationality' state. I experience it as a struggle, at times with the feeling state winning over 'Rationality' and bringing itself to the surface, becoming executive.

These are normal and appropriate processes. I would not want to be in 'Rationality' all the time. That is a sterile and cold state that is useful for thinking, and for a break from being overexposed with feelings, but it is a state where I do not experience love, and awe, and wonder. I want to be able to bring out my fragile, feeling states when it is safe, and I want to be able to use other states when it is appropriate. If a feeling state has unprocessed material it is appropriate for it to come to the surface so some resolution can be made. Knowing your states does not mean that this resolution is painless or easy.

I have been able to better function, and better enjoy life following my improved understanding of my ego state map. Being familiar with my states has given me a personal understanding that I appreciate and has given me a power of choice that I did not previously enjoy. I am better able to 'feel' when it is safe, and 'protect' when it is not. It has allowed me to feel more deeply, and it has enriched my life.

3.3.1 Ego State Mapping

Ego state mapping is the process of learning which ego states a person has, the roles of the states, which states know other states and the nature of their communication, and how to call the individual states to the executive so they can be used at the most preferred times. Hypnosis is necessary to get a good ego state map, because without hypnosis only the commonly used surface states can be mapped.

Therapeutic interventions for the resolution of trauma or to improve communication between states will involve a degree of ego state mapping, as good notes should be kept with information concerning all ego states contacted. These interventions differ from ego state mapping sessions, as they entail contacting ego states only to achieve the immediate goals of therapy. There is not an effort to produce a more complete map of the client's ego state structure. Ego state mapping is to provide the client with information that may be useful in achieving higher performance, more satisfaction, and greater enjoyment. It is important to note that during the process of mapping trauma and/or poor communication between states may become evident. If this occurs, clients who have asked specifically for mapping sessions should be asked if they wish to extend the scope of the sessions to therapeutic intervention.

It appears to be impossible to do a self-mapping. We need the assistance of another hypnotherapist to discover our states, at least our underlying states.

During a mapping session, discussion with each state is limited mainly to 1) role, 2) name, 3) knowledge other states, 4) attitude toward other states, and 5) willingness to help either in communication or role.

The client needs to decide the preferred scope of the ego state mapping (see section 3.3.5). Does the client want a mapping of mainly surface states, or is a more complete mapping of surface and underlying states preferred? This decision will entail a balancing between time and money, and level of self-awareness desired.

1. *Role.*

   The first step in ego state mapping is to gain access to ego states in one of the ways described in Chapter 2 above. It is helpful to have large, blank sheets of paper available. When talking with an ego state first ask about its function or role. This gives useful information for ego state naming.

2. *Name.*

   Next ask the ego state what you can call it. It is a good idea to write down and circle the name it prefers. This makes it easy to quickly locate the name on a page that will become full of words, lines, and arrows. It is not unusual for a state to have some difficulty choosing a name and it may be necessary to suggest a name yourself, but always check that the name you choose is acceptable with the state with which you are speaking. For example, if the role of the state is to tidy and clean, you might ask the state if you could call it 'Cleaner'. It is important to get a name so you can call the state to the executive again, and so there is a reference to the state for communication with other states. You will be able to ask other states if they know 'Cleaner'.

   Always give the state the first opportunity to name itself, and do not assign a name to a state without first checking that the state is happy to accept the name. Occasionally a state will give itself a negative name, such as 'Dummy'. When this happens I attempt to see if there is a less negative name that the state will be happy with, but if the state is reluctant to change the name, I will accept the negative name. In therapy it is often the case that a state that first gives itself a negative sounding name, later wants to change the name to something more positive to reflect its change in role, or function.

3. *Knowledge of other states.*

   Most ego states communicate frequently with one or more other states. It is useful in mapping ego states to discover which states each ego state knows and communicates with. "What other states do you know?" can be a revealing question. Another technique is to ask the state that is executive if it knows states you have already discovered. I like to draw a pencil line between the circled names of the states when they know each other. There will often be clusters of states that know each other well, and work together, and they may be quite separate from other states or clusters of states. There are often surface and underlying states that have no knowledge of the existence of some underlying ego states.

4. *Attitude toward other states.*
    Along the pencil line that connects states that know or communicate together I write comments about how the states think and feel about each other. Above the line I put an arrow in one direction and below the line I put an arrow in the other direction. This allows me to know the feeling of each state toward the other. For example, if the state, 'Protector', dislikes 'Hedonist', above the line I would make a note of this with the arrow pointing from 'Protector' to 'Hedonist'. Below the line the arrow would point in the opposite direction with comments on the attitude 'Hedonist' holds toward 'Protector'.

5. *Willingness to help.*
    An important part of mapping is discovering how the different states would like to be helpful. It is useful information for the client to learn about a state that has skills in assertiveness so that state can interact with people when the client calls it to the executive. A wise state may be asked to call upon either the state that can be assertive or a state that can show more anger, depending on the situational need. Ego state mapping can inform clients of their potential and give them the awareness needed to reach toward it.

3.3.2   Advantages of Knowing Your States

There are several advantages people gain from learning about their ego states. A number of my clients have said they feel much better in just knowing who they are and why they are the way they are. When we experience our own states and understand what each state feels it is a self-revelation. Some clients have said they thought they were crazy, the way their mood changed in a seemingly random fashion. When they learn their states and where their states come from, and the role of each state, it makes sense to them. They feel empowered and better able to be in control in their life. The following section will deal with how learning our ego states can increase personal development, and our ability to enjoy life.

3.3.3   *Personal Development with Ego State Therapy*

Knowing our states can benefit our personal development in several ways. Some of the assets include:

- We can become assertive at appropriate times.
- We can be angry at appropriate times.
- We can be confident in speaking.
- We can safely experience the emotional depths of childhood, regardless of our age.
- We can feel love.
- We can face criticism without feeling abused.
- We can be our logical self when it is appropriate.
- We can be our party self when it is appropriate.
- We can experience better physical health.

A hug while in a fragile, child state can be an extraordinary experience. It is felt and appreciated deeply. A hug while in an intellectual state feels cold and uneasy. Imagine what it would be like having to live in a single ego state. Consider a hypothetical person, Paul, who is stuck in a head/rational state. Paul responds to everything rationally. There is no evident confusion over choice, since there is only the rational choice. There are no evident feelings of joy, fear, love, or hate. There is no excitement or feelings of awe and wonder. There is just "getting down to business", just evenness, just the affect of an android. There are some Paul's out there who have learned to stay in one or two states almost all the time, to the detriment of their ability to enjoy living.

What defines us is our feelings, our ability to experience love, awe, wonder, fear, and even hate. We are affective people in a wonderfully affective world. Too often we lose the ability to be a child, or to think of what we want, rather than what we "should" have. We are made up of a large number of ego states with a wide variety of potentials. Our most enjoyable states are the child states. It takes a combination of courage and wisdom to access them readily.

Many of us learn, as we age, that it is easier to stay away from some of the more fragile child states that have the capacity to really get excited, to love, and to be amazed, but also have the capacity to hurt, and fear. We not only have these fragile inner states, but we have states whose role it is to protect them; states that are a bit hard and crusty, with a shell, or a sharp tongue. Learning our states allows us the ability to allow a fragile child state into the executive to experience the 'wow' of a hug, to experience love, awe, taste, and more when it is safe. A wise state can be called upon to act as the traffic director to see if the time is safe to allow the child state into the executive, and to decide when the child state should be protected by calling out a tougher, protector state. The goal is to experience powerful feelings, without feeling exposed, or overexposed.

We can learn that it is safe to call out a fragile child state (all child states are not fragile) when we are with someone who we can trust. It is important to learn to expose fragile states only when it is safe, and allow the protector states to do their job when it is not safe. It would not be good to expose a fragile state to someone who would likely hurt it. This would make it more difficult for that state to become executive the next time. The more a state is hurt, the less it is willing to come out. This is why it is useful to use a wise state to determine the safety of allowing a fragile child state to come to the executive.

I have a state that is so fragile that I have learned to call it out only when I am with someone with whom I have great trust, and then only when my eyes are closed. When I have great trust and get a loving hug I can call this state into the executive, and the experience is incredible. It feels like a very young state (started when I was young), so I have named it 'Infant'. If I stay in 'Infant' and open my eyes I can easily feel overexposed. My wise state understands this and only calls infant out when it is safe to feel that wonderful flow of love from someone I can trust. If I am with people whose purpose and/or honesty are something I question, my wise state calls out some a nice hard, crusty, assertive state that can handle hardship; a state with well-oiled feathers that can protect my fragile parts.

3.3.4 Self Talk for Health: Experiencing Better Physical Health

Common colds were my experience about twice a year. It has been many years since I have had a cold. The ego state technique for this is simple. I call it, "Self Talk for Health". When I feel a cold coming, I sit in an easy chair and place myself into a light state of hypnosis. I then ask the general question aimed at the state that has chosen for me to have a cold, "What is it that you need from me so I won't have to have this cold?" Then I listen for the answer. It is not important for me to know which state may answer. Of course I don't hear an outside voice that could be picked up with a microphone, but I am definitely aware of an answer. It is usually something like, "Get more sleep", or "Eat more", or sometimes, "Eat a meal with a lot of chili". I'm not sure why chili, but I do it. Sometimes the answer is, "Take time to de-stress ..." about some issue that is occurring in my life. Sometimes it is a combination of the above, or something different. Occasionally, I have negotiated, "I need one more late night, and then I promise I will get lots of sleep for the next few days." Usually, what is asked is easy and I merely say, "OK, I will do what you asked. Will you help me not have this cold?" I get an answer. It has worked every time.

To those who have not worked with ego states this technique may sound outside reasonable practice. Paul Federn (1952) defined sanity as being able to tell the difference between the internal and the external. This activity is working with the internal, with the ego states. Most often I do not make an attempt to determine which states are communicating together. What I am most interested in is acquiring the desired result.

A benefit of the "Self Talk for Health" technique is that after learning it the person can continue to use it without the aid of a therapist, and it can be applied to a variety of health concerns. It is especially good for headaches, colds, flu, and backache. It is most useful when applied at the earliest warning signs of the physical ailment.

Recently, a woman came to me who had participated in one of my workshops. She had chosen use "Self Talk for Health" with her premenstrual condition. PMS had bothered her for many years, and after applying this ego state technique she had been PMS free for over a year.

In order for it to be used, it is important that those using it know self-hypnosis, and have an understanding of ego states and their function. While scientific investigation has not confirmed its efficacy it shows promise, not only in the above areas, but also in many other areas such as fertility and endometriosis.

3.3.5 *How many States to know?*

Ego state mapping will probably never result in all ego states being mapped or known. It is up to the individual to decide how extensive a mapping is desired. Most of the surface states, the states that often become executive, and some underlying states may be mapped in a single session. A single session of ego state mapping will generally result in the client and the hypnotherapist becoming familiar with 5 to 15 states. Becoming familiar with this number of states, especially with common surface states, can be enriching for the client. We have a much larger number of states.

Some clients will wish to gain a more full understanding of their ego state structure, and learn about their underlying states. These underlying states affect us occasionally, and often possess assets from which we seldom gain benefit. Learning about these states will give the client a more full understanding of his or her personality, strengths, and resources. It will also provide the client with a rather detailed history of experiences, since allowing underlying states expression brings to the surface experiences of those childhood states. It is important to note that the memories of any ego state may not be totally accurate. This is true for both surface states and underlying states, as is illustrated by witnesses' varying accounts of an auto accident.

A more complete ego state mapping will take several sessions, especially if issue processing is undertaken. This type of mapping will result in the client gaining a keen understanding of self and personal history. It will allow the person to be more fully functioning, even when issue processing is not undertaken. This more complete mapping results in the same kind of awareness that traditional psychoanalysts hope to achieve during the course of analysis. Ego state mapping allows this result in a few sessions, while psychoanalysis requires numerous sessions over a few years.

It is not unusual for trauma to be uncovered during ego state mapping, regardless of the detail of the mapping. It is incumbent upon the therapist, when this occurs, to ask the client if he or she would like to process that trauma. When a client has come for mapping, and has not indicated a desire to work on issues a verbal contract is needed before issue processing is undertaken. Often the mapping may proceed and the client can decide after the session about returning to work on the issues that may have become evident. Occasionally, a prime opportunity exists during a mapping session to process issues. The client may be asked immediately if this is something that would be preferred. It should be noted that bringing forth a trauma and not processing it would leave the client feeling closer to the experience of the trauma. It is preferred to process trauma, rather than to leave it unprocessed, although this should always be the decision of the client.

Chapter 4

Applications of
Ego State Therapy

The most common applications of this therapy relate to the goals of finding and resolving trauma, improving the nature of internal communication among states, and improving the client's knowledge and accessibility of states. This section investigates some specific applications where Ego State Therapy is powerful. The applications selected for inclusion were chosen for illustration and should not be considered a complete listing of possible applications for this therapy. Ego State Therapy is a relatively new and evolving psychotherapy. As it further develops and becomes available to more therapists its nature and use will broaden accordingly.

4.1   Alleviating Psychosomatic Symptoms

One of the indicators of *dissociative identity disorder* (multiple personality) is a frequent headache. This is not to say that a person who has frequent headaches is a multiple. There are several indicators, but the struggle between alters (multiple personalities) does often result in headache, especially when two alters are struggling for the executive (to be the one out). Likewise, when a person with normal ego states experiences a struggle between internal states headache is often the result. This is an example of a psychosomatic symptom caused by ego states.

Gainer (1993) reported a patient who, with hypnosis, identified an ego state that after collecting childhood pain, transferred the pain to a physical symptom by developing Reflex Sympathetic Dystrophy in an arm. This is a syndrome that is normally progressive and can result in the need for amputation. Ego State Therapy techniques resolved the child pain and facilitated a complete remission. It is interesting that the patient had at least three ego states that did not experience the reflex sympathetic dystrophy and when they were executive (prior to the remission) the symptoms were moderated or disappeared, only to return when other ego states assumed the executive. The remission was not evident in all ego states until the childhood issues had been resolved.

Some physiological symptoms are caused by underlying ego states and some symptoms are purely organic in origin. The symptoms of stress and the decay of a tooth are obvious examples of each. An individual may also be genetically predisposed to develop a physical symptom and underlying ego states may play a role in increasing or lessening the occurrence of that symptom becoming manifested.

Ego State Therapy can be useful in three ways to assess and dispel or moderate physical symptoms:

1. Discovery of a psychosomatic connection, if one exists.
2. Discovery of the cause.
3. Resolution of the cause.

4.2   Ego State Therapy in the Control of Pain

There is an adage in business, "You never get something for nothing." A similar cliché is, "If it sounds too good to be true, it probably is." These old clichés rightly apply to the use of hypnosis for pain control. Hypnosis has been used as an analgesic for many years. The Scottish sergeant, James Esdaile, performed numerous medical operations on hypnotized patients before the advent of chemical pain relievers (Emmerson, 1987). Hypnosis continues to be used to assist patients to either feel no pain, or reduce the experience of pain. There is no doubt that the use of hypnosis can result in altering the patient's conscious experience of pain. There is concern about the internal dynamic at work that facilitates this altered experience. How is it that a hypnotized person can watch a pin go through his or her hand and experience no feeling? The nerves are being cut and displaced. Signals are being sent to the brain. What happens to the pain?

It is important for hypnotherapists who work with pain to have a clear understanding of the internal dynamic of pain control. The experiences a patient reports are experiences of the executive ego state. Other ego states that often become executive will share memories of those experiences also, since the communication between these states is very good. Underlying ego states that rarely, or never, become executive may also experience through sensory perception, although often our conscious, executive state is unaware of this. This has been demonstrated by scientific experiments (Hilgard, 1975; Watkins and Watkins, 1990).

Hilgard (1975) found that he could suggest to hypnotized subjects that they would not be able to hear any noise, and they would experience total hypnotic deafness, until a cessation cue was given. During these experiments he found that states he called 'hidden observers' could hear and respond, while the conscious subject could not. After the experiment the conscious state would have no memory of this hidden observer state that was able to hear during the experiment. He further found that these hidden observers could feel pain when the subject reported feeling no pain.

Watkins and Watkins (1990) described an experiment on anesthesia and hypnosis, "One subject kept the hypnotically anesthetized right hand in the ice water five times as long as he did the unanesthetized left hand and then developed a severe stomach ache. The pain had apparently been displaced from the hand to the stomach" (p. 7). The Watkins confirmed this by speaking directly to the dissociated ego state that had experienced and displaced the pain. This state that had felt the pain was quite upset over the experience.

Pain, anger, and frustration can be held in subconscious ego states, and these toxic feelings can result in problematic emotional or medical symptom etiology. Gainer's (1993) patient, through hypnosis, identified an ego state that after collecting childhood pain chose to get rid of the pain by developing Reflex Sympathetic Dystrophy in her arm. As reported above, Ego State Therapy facilitated a complete remission. Watkins (1990) reported a patient in whom the arm pain of an underlying ego state was transferred by another ego state to stomach pain.

The importance here is that when hypnosis is used to eliminate or reduce the experience of pain, we may be merely transferring that pain from a conscious state to an unconscious state, a state that may cause problems for the patient because of this pain experience. When a state experiences pain, there needs to be an understanding, an acceptance, a resolution, otherwise the experience may be carried as an unresolved trauma. Every state needs resolution.

Pain may be the result of a physical cause or a psychological (ego state related) cause, and these two types of pain each require specific consideration.

PAIN RESULTING FROM A PHYSICAL CAUSE

If the cause of pain is not psychological, it is physical. Pain resulting from a purely physical cause may result from something like dental work. If the pain results from a physical cause, hypnosis for the relief of this pain may result in non-executive ego states taking on the pain, and thus causing physical or emotional symptom etiology later. Pharmacological blocking of this type of pain should result in no direct psychological issues. This means that a person who uses hypnosis when a tooth is being drilled so pain is not experienced at a conscious level, may well be experiencing that pain on a subconscious level, and that experience may become problematic for the person later. If, though, Novocain is used to block the pain from being received in the brain, then there is no storage of psychological pain.

Consider the person who visits a dentist and receives hypnosis in order to experience no pain during dental work. When the dentist drills, pain signals are being sent to the brain. The conscious, executive, ego state does not experience the pain, but an underlying ego state does experience the pain. Without ego state work, it is impossible to determine, "Where goes the ouch?" (Watkins and Watkins, 1990), or what problems the patient may later experience. If the underlying ego state that experienced the pain did not understand where the pain came from, or did not accept the role of experiencing the pain, an unresolved trauma can be the result. A major emphasis of this book is that ego states need resolution for what is feared or not understood. When resolution is not achieved the unresolved state can cause the person to feel generally unsettled, can cause neurotic symptoms, or can cause unwanted physiological symptoms.

It is therefore normally not recommended to use hypnosis for the direct elimination of physically caused pain. If it is important to use hypnosis for the relief of the symptoms of this type of pain, it is recommended that such work be followed with accessing the ego state(s) that took on the pain, so an appropriate therapeutic release may be facilitated. Ego state work prior to a physically painful experience may prepare an underlying state that will voluntarily experience the pain with an understanding that it is helping the client by keeping the pain from the conscious, executive state. Even when this arrangement is made it is recommended to revisit this state after the experience to make sure no unresolved feelings exist.

When a person experiences pain and is able to vent that pain to the external world (let others know about the pain, and feel expressed and understood), then normally no 'pain baggage' accrues. One hypnotic way of assisting clients with the symptoms of pain is using a dual ego state awareness. This dissociation allows the pain to be felt consciously by one state, while a second conscious state has no experience of pain. The person will have a full awareness of the pain, but it will seem like the pain "is not mine".

PAIN RESULTING FROM A PSYCHOLOGICAL CAUSE

If the pain results from an ego state origin (a psychological cause), then hypnosis for the symptoms of this pain may inhibit and frustrate the ego state that caused the pain, and other physical or emotional symptom etiology may follow. Hypnosis addressing the cause of the pain (the ego state causing the pain) should result in a relief of pain with no adverse effects. Research on menstrual migraine indicated that underlying ego states often cause menstrual migraine (Emmerson and Farmer, 1996). When these ego states were negotiated with the average number of migraine days per month in the sample went from 12.2 to 2.5.

It may be possible to determine if the cause of a pain, such as a migraine, is physical or psychological. This can often be determined by speaking with the ego states, seeing if a state takes responsibility for the pain, and seeing if this state can turn the pain on and off. It is important for the client to be in a medium to deep hypnotic state. The client should be able to switch easily between states before attempting to determine if a pain has an ego state cause. An example of a request to learn more about a pain is, "I would like to speak with at state that knows something about (for example) where the migraines come from. Is there a state that causes the migraines? I would very much like to talk with that state, or a state that knows about that state please. Just say I'm here when you are ready to speak."

A second method of tracing the possible origin of a pain is to ask the hypnotized client to experience the pain (this can normally be accomplished easily by using imagery to place the client at a time and place when the pain was experienced). While the client is experiencing the pain, ask about any associated emotional feelings, then use the affect bridge to go to the origin of the pain. If probing of this type, using both methods while the client is in a good hypnotic state and is easily switching between states, results in no states coming forward with information concerning the pain, then it is more likely that the pain results from a physiological cause.

Pharmacological blocking of pain stemming from an ego state cause may inhibit and frustrate the ego state that caused the pain, and other physical or emotional symptom etiology may follow. A probable example of this is 'rebound headaches' (Cady and Farmer, 1993) that sometimes result from pharmacological treatment for migraine. Therefore, it is not good to attempt to remove a psychologically caused pain with pharmacology, or with hypnosis unless the cause for the pain symptom is addressed. If an unresolved ego state is giving a person pain, the resolution needs to be addressed, not the pain symptom.

WORKING WITH EGO STATES WITH PAIN WITH A PSYCHOLOGICAL CAUSE

Ego state negotiation is necessary to alter the internal dynamics when psychosomatic pain is present. An *internal group therapy* (Caul, 1984) can be used to detoxify these troubled, subconscious ego states. Everything happens for a reason. When an ego state causes the client to experience pain there is some reason behind it. The logic of this causal ego state may be faulty, confused, or angry. It is important to deal with the ego state that is causing the pain, with respect and understanding, and to present an appreciation of the power of the state. It is important to get the state to want to cooperate for the good of the person. A good way to do this is to remind the state that it was born to help the client, and that you (the therapist) want to help the client and in order to do so, you need the help of this powerful state. Additionally, it is normally helpful to appeal to the state by talking about how 'it must not feel very good being disliked by other states', and about how good it might feel to be liked and accepted by the other states. Often this approach at first meet with statements such as, "I don't care what they think", or "They would never like me". Relentless, diplomatic negotiation can bring this state back into the family of states as a respected and appreciated member. As this occurs the state will soften and become appreciative of the new acceptance.

Ego states that cause physical pain often report that it is all they know to do. It is important for them to take on a new role that is appropriate so they can cease the role of 'Pain Giver'. Sometimes they will be able to give guidance in relation to what their new role might be, and sometimes the therapists can think of possibilities and check to see if the state would be happy with the new role. The scope of these roles relies only on creativity. A role that pain giving ego states are often willing to accept is that of appropriate pain giver. The ego state, through negotiation, agrees to accept a lesser role and give some of its to a different, specified state that can use it appropriately. With its remaining energy the pain giving state gives the client pain only when it may protect the client from harm. If the client gets too close to a flame the state may give the client a pain so the client will not move any closer, or if there is something physical that requires attention the state can make sure that the client receives enough pain to notice and react appropriately. This role of appropriate pain giver can be presented as an important role that the other states can appreciate. The state that may have been isolated from some other states can rejoin the family of states.

It is a good procedure to encourage the other states to communicate with the state that had caused pain, both during the negotiation process and at its conclusion. These other states will often, at first, say things like, "He will never do anything but cause pain." A good response is, "But if he was to cause pain only if it was really needed to draw attention for safety or healing, would you accept him doing that important job?" When these states agree that they will cooperate and accept the state in its new role, especially when they express this to the state, the negotiation is near its conclusion. When this agreement is made the therapist can say, "That's great. I wonder if you can say to 'name of pain causing state' that you will appreciate him in this new role. You can talk with him silently about it now. (pause) Tell me what happened."

Continue to check with all states involved during any ego state negotiation. Treat each with respect and do not get discouraged when states say, "never". It is amazing how positive they can become during the process of negotiation.

4.3   *Couples Counseling*

When two people want to maintain a good relationship or have difficulty in just keeping their relationship going, they sometimes seek help in couples counseling. Couples may want to heal a damaged relationship or enhance a relationship that promises more. Ego State Therapy helps couples by assisting them in communication and in awareness, both self awareness and awareness of the other partner. Ego State Therapy can also help a relationship by individually helping partners in a relationship clear away their own traumas and their own internal ego state communication problems that might otherwise interfere in the relationship.

Relationship problems can arise from various difficulties. Three major areas of difficulty in relationships are differences in ideas or philosophy, problems in communication, and individual problems a partner may experience that may impinge on the relationship. While Ego State Therapy is not an intervention that is aimed toward changing ideas or philosophy, it still can be useful to look at some differences in ideas that can cause problems in a relationship. Examples of differences in ideas include the following.

- Religious beliefs – These can range from major differences in basic beliefs to differences in how, or how often, a belief should be practiced.
- Children – Do both partners want children? If so, how many? How should children be raised?
- Roles – How are the required tasks divided?
- Money – Where does the money come from? How much should be spent and on what? How are the decisions made for spending or saving money?
- Other relationships – What kinds of other relationships are acceptable? How much time should be spent interacting as a couple?
- Holidays and free time – How should time be spent (e.g., mountains, cafés, shopping, at home)?
- Extended family – What is the role of the extended family in the relationship, and how much time is spent with them?
- Vocation – How important is the vocation of each partner? Whose vocation dictates the living location of the couple?
- Sexual issues – The frequency and nature of sexual activity, and what is acceptable within the relationship (provocative movies, shows, clothes, flirtations, other partners).
- Health and fitness – Diet and exercise. What foods should be eaten and what body fitness should be maintained. What legal (e.g., caffeine, nicotine, alcohol) or non-legal drugs (e.g., marijuana, cocaine, heroin), if any, are acceptable?
- Disclosure – How much information is shared with the partner? How honest or trustworthy is the relationship?
- Step-families – Relationships with ex-partners or stepchildren can generate difficult issues.

This is only a partial list of idea issues from which couples can have difficulty. Looking at the list a person can wonder how any two people are ever able to maintain a relationship. Many do. One of the ways they do, when they cannot agree on ideas, is by communicating. Good communication is imperative for a good relationship.

A common problem couples have in communicating relates to the states from which each is communicating at a given time. It is important for each person to be able to express fully, and to feel heard and understood. In order for this to happen the state that is executive must be able to speak with a state of their partner that can hear and understand what needs to be said.

An angry state of one partner should not be executive at the same time as a defensive state of the other partner. This would result in the angry state feeling unheard and resented, and often feeling even more angry, and the defensive state of the other partner feeling attacked. When one partner is speaking from an angry state the other partner needs to be in a more removed, intellectual, understanding state in order to hear what is being said, process it, and show understanding without getting upset. This intellectual state does not have to agree with what the angry state is saying, but it does need to be able to show an understanding of the other partner's perspective.

A state with pent-up feelings needs to be able to release those feelings, and if the pent-up feelings are held toward a partner, to resolve those feelings it is best if the feelings can be expressed to the partner. Expressing the feelings and feeling heard is like letting the steam out of a pressure cooker.

Couples counseling can be thought of as a four-phase process, the individual phase, the co-learning phase, the negotiation phase, and the practice phase. It is not necessary for all four phases to reach completion in order for a relationship to improve, but until all phases have been completed the potential of the relationship cannot be realized.

Prior to the first phase it is important to make sure that both partners want the relationship to continue. Unless both want to invest work on the relationship it may be that some form of separation counseling is most useful. Given that both partners want an improved relationship, ego state couples counseling normally takes a minimum of seven sessions. In the first session of counseling the two partners will meet together with the therapist to describe and define their problem. During this session the process of ego state couples counseling can be explained. The individual phase will take a minimum of two sessions (one for each client), and this phase may take a number of sessions depending on the needs of the clients.

The remaining three phases may be completed with in a single session for each, or they may take multiple sessions, depending on the couple. A final session will follow the forth phase in order to make sure that the couple is ready to continue to use their states together in a positive way. Couples counseling sessions generally follow the following timetable, although the depending on the couple the length of the phases (especially the individual phase) may vary.

- **Week 1:** Definition session: The partners come in together to define the problem and indicate a desire to invest time and effort into the relationship.
- **Weeks 2–3:** (or multiple sessions depending on need), Individual Phase: These are individual sessions.
- **Week 4:** (depending on length of Individual Phase), Co-learning Phase: The partners come in together.
- **Week 5:** (depending of preceding phases), Negotiation Phase: The partners come in together.
- **Week 6:** (depending on preceding phases), Practice Phase: The partners come in together. It may be that one or both partners feel a need at one of these later phases to return for further individual work.
- **Week 7:** (depending on preceding phases), Follow-up Session: The partners come in together. This session is to make sure the couple is ready to continue on their own. It may best occur at least two weeks following the Practice Phase.

PHASE 1 – INDIVIDUAL PHASE
This is the only phase in ego state couples counseling that requires the use of hypnosis. It is difficult for most people to learn about underlying states without hypnosis, and how these states can greatly add to the richness of a relationship. The ego state mapping (see section 3.3) of each partner is a necessary step in couples counseling. Each partner needs to learn personal states in order to be able to call upon and use those states at various times in couples communication.

Each partner should resolve individual traumas (see section 3.1), and internal ego state communication problems (see section 3.2).

Internal traumas can result in spurious or neurotic reactions within the relationship that cannot be resolved by focusing merely on the communication between partners. For example, if unresolved anger exists concerning a parental relationship while a partner was a child, reactions toward a partner may be more of a reflection of the unresolved anger toward a parent than a reflection of true feelings about the partner. If the internal communication within a partner does not allow an acceptance of self, that partner will not be able to respond appropriately within a relationship.

PHASE 2 – CO-LEARNING PHASE

Couples, with the help of the therapist, should learn each other's states, along with the talents and weaknesses of each state. It is not enough for each partner to know many of their own states. The partners also need to know and appreciate the states of their partners. What is important is that they learn as many ego states as practical, both their own and their partners, while in counseling. They need to understand the importance of no state being dismissed and left out of the communication process. When each partner learns their own states and the states of their partners they will begin to understand why it is important for some states to avoid each other, and others to prefer to talk together. It does not help a state with pent-up feelings to be met by a state feeling resentment. The state that feels the resentment, likewise, does not like to feel attacked by feeling the anger of the partner. By the end of this phase partners will begin to understand the importance of one state asking to speak directly to a specific state of their partner (e.g., "My adolescent state would like to talk with your nurturing state.").

PHASE 3 – NEGOTIATION PHASE

Partners should learn during the negotiation phase that the four steps to problem resolution are:

1. Releasing/listening
2. Talking
3. Bargaining
4. Resolving

They should learn which of their states are best suited for each step. Different ego states may be needed for each of these four steps, or the same state may be used in multiple steps. For example, John may need to release from an angry state while Julie listens from an intellectual understanding state (releasing/listening step). Julie may need to release from a frustrated state while John listens from a nurturing state (releasing/listening step). Both John and Julie may prefer to discuss the issue (talking step) from reflective states. Julie may want to use her assertiveness state in the bargaining step, while John may prefer to use his business state during this step. John or Julie may decide to use the same state in the resolution step that they chose for the bargaining step, or one or both may wish to use a different state.

The states that are chosen by each partner for the fours steps of problem resolution are only first examples. As their communication process evolves post couples therapy they will spontaneously refine which states can best talk with the states of their partner, and at which times. The increased self awareness and awareness and respect of the partner will help the communication process to positively evolve. Prior to this type of therapy it is easy for a partner to believe that the most difficult state of a partner is that partner. Learning about how the personality is structured allows each partner to know of the other that while there are states there that may be having difficulty with aspects of the relationship, there are also states that have much love, acceptance and respect.

During the negotiation phase the therapist should speak with each of the states (of each partner) that will likely be communicating during the four steps of problem resolution. Agreement should be made with each state that will be playing a role in problem resolution. For example, the therapist might asked an intellectual state of one partner, "Are you willing to talk with Amy's anger state when she is angry about something and needs to express it?" If a state is not willing to take up a role in this process, a different state should be sought that can and would like to participate in this process (see section 4.5.2).

The negotiation phase does not have to be inclusive of all the combinations of interactions the states of the partners will want to enjoy together. It could not be. Partners will continue to learn what interactions work best. They will be able to be creative.

PHASE 4 – PRACTICE PHASE

Couples should bring out real life issues and practice switching and using the states that are most helpful in communication and resolution. Notes from the first session can be referred to in order to make sure issues are practiced that have been problematic to the couple in the past. During this process the therapist needs to help each partner make sure the preferred state is executive. If a reactive state jumps into the executive prematurely, the therapist should assure that state that it is important for it to be heard, and that it will have an opportunity to speak before the discussion is finished. It can be assured that not only will it have an opportunity to speak, but that it will be able to speak to a state that will be able to hear it. If the partners are able to follow though the problem resolution process in counseling, they will likely be able to follow though on their own, given the will to do so. They need to be clear that issues may arise after leaving therapy that will necessitate creativity on their part and they may need to call on states that were not a part of training in therapy.

4.3.1   Bringing Relationships to a Higher Level: The Enhanced Relationship

Ego state techniques can bring a relationship to a higher level of enjoyment and fulfillment. It can help a relationship with normal levels of communication to high levels of intimacy. Couples who have resolved communication problems may want to continue to achieve enhanced communication and enjoyment in the relationship. Couples who already have good communication may want to use Ego State Therapy to achieve this higher level of enjoyment in their relationship.

Healing destructive communication patterns requires that certain ego states of one partner should not attempt to talk with specific ego states of the other partner. An angry state of one partner and a defensive state of the other partner should not attempt to communicate directly with each other. The manner to achieve an enhanced relationship is the bringing together ego states that can, not just communicate to resolve issues, but can fully enjoy each other.

One partner may have an ego state that feels fragile and in real need of love and hugs, while the other partner may have a state that truly enjoys nurturing. When these two states can be executive at the same time both partners can enjoy deep emotional closeness. The fragile state may have learned to hide in the relationship in fear of a disapproving state of the partner that could bring pain. The fragile state will learn it is safe to come to the executive when the partners are able to learn the importance of respecting each other's states and using the states for a higher enjoyment of the relationship.

The phases to an enhanced relationship are the same as those to heal a destructive relationship, the individual phase, the co-learning phase, the negotiation phase, and the practice phase. A relationship can be improved without a completion of all four phases, but the potential of the relationship cannot be met. For example, a past trauma may inhibit a closeness in one aspect of the relationship, but partners may still be able to bring out states that enjoy each other.

Relationships are enhanced when partners learn not only their own states, but also the states of their partners. They are better able to understand and respect each other. They can be proud of the parts of their partners that they now can ask to come to the executive for special communication (e.g., "My child part would love a hug from your nurturing part." Or "This tastes fantastic. Can 'Hedonist' have a taste of this?").

The practice phase of enhancement counseling can involve practice in the counseling office and at home. It is important that each partner to learn to bring different ego states to the executive in the counseling office to insure the technique has been learned. It is often quite easy for a client to bring an ego state to the executive once it has been talked with directly during counseling. This is true even for an underlying ego state. The home practice can be private and need not be reported in detail to the therapist. It is only important for the therapist to be able to give assistance if the partners are having difficulty with the process of selecting and bringing to the executive ego states that most want to enjoy each other.

It may be the case that a critical or pent-up state has a need to be heard before a nurturing or fragile state can enjoy the relationship. Partners should learn that each state must be respected, and that by fulfilling the needs of each state, every state can more fully enjoy the relationship.

4.4   Reducing Depression and Anger

Ego State Therapy provides a process of resolving residual trauma and improving internal communication between states so the person can feel more integrated, positive, and self-accepting. Even when the dealing with depression and anger are not the primary goal of the client, the process that reduces trauma and improves internal communication necessarily lowers depression and anger. The ego state menstrual migraine study previously referred to (Emmerson and Farmer, 1996) was aimed to determine the effectiveness of Ego State Therapy for the symptoms of menstrual migraine. Depression levels of the participants were measured (both before and after treatment) using the MMPI-2 and the Beck Depression Scale, with both scales indicating a significant reduction in levels of depression. The MMPI-2 further indicated significant reductions in anger using pre-post testing.

4.4.1   Depression

Depression is often the result of one or more states feeling isolated, misunderstood, and hopeless. These states need to be able to express their needs directly, to feel heard, understood, and respected. They may need to learn new roles that they can respect and that can be respected by other ego states. Depression is the result of ego states that have and hold onto energy, but refuse to use it or allow it to be used by other states. Holding this energy along with negative feelings, especially feelings of loss, prevents the client from being able to properly engage with the outside world.

A woman with a 'flirty' ego state that enjoys flirting and gaining the positive attention of others may experience a severe loss of energy when a severe burn scars her face. This ego state may feel hopeless and unable to fulfill its mission of flirting and gaining positive feedback and appreciation from other people. The whole person can feel less energy, if the flirty ego state hangs onto the energy it was once able to use, rather than either finding new ways of using it, or transferring it to other states. Talking with an intellectual ego state about the problem will not help 'flirty' and will do little to restructure the energy usage in the family of states. 'Flirty' would need to be addressed directly. Ego state negotiation needs to result in 'flirty' taking on a role that matches the energy she maintains. She may wish to give or trade some energy to other states, and there are always states that would like more. It is important for 'Flirty' to feel positive about any new role, or the transfer of energy. Ego state negotiation can be used to facilitate this process (see section 3.2.1).

4.4.2 Anger

Ego State Therapy can assist in working with two types of problems concerning anger. A client can have a problem in 'not releasing' anger, and can also have a problem in 'how anger is released'. Holding onto anger tends to create more psychological distress internally, while inappropriately expressing anger tends to create more sociological problems externally. These, in turn, can result in psychological anxiety.

Hanging on to, or holding, anger can result in passive-aggressive behavior, in panic attacks, or in other psychological or physical distress. Ego state negotiation can result in ego states that have learned to hold anger, learning to communicate better with an assertive state so the anger can be released in an appropriate fashion. It is important that every state be satisfied with any arrangement of role reassignment.

A client of mine once presented with the problem of loosing his temper. The incident that finally convinced him to come to therapy for this problem concerned his pet dog. My client arrived home one afternoon already very angry concerning another person, when he discovered his dog had made a wet spot on the carpet. My client's anger increased and he started yelling at, and hitting, his dog. The dog, becoming distressed, made another wet spot on the carpet. My client became incensed and threw his dog off the balcony. The dog was killed. This incident appropriately scared my client, and he came to therapy. During the initial interview I asked him if there was anything that helped calm his anger. He replied that there used to be. "What", I asked. He replied, "My dog".

It is imperative to talk with the state that needs to change. It would have done little good for me to just talk with my client about the state that could get angry and then express that anger inappropriately. Before hypnosis I asked for detail concerning the incident when the dog was killed. What time of day was it? What were you wearing? What did you dog look like when you got home? Where was he? What did the wet spot look like? Could you smell it? This type of questioning can help the client to return to the ego state that needs to change. After hypnosis I used this information to the executive the ego state that was angry.

We discovered that this state felt it not only had a right to be angry, but that it had a responsibility to be angry when things did not go well in life. Ego state negotiation resulted in this state agreeing to allow a wiser state to determine when anger should be expressed overtly as rage, or when anger should be expressed overtly as assertive behavior. It was decided that rage could be appropriate if he were physically attacked by person or beast, and needed rage to defend himself. It was also decided that an assertive expression of feelings with statements such as, "I am really angry right now", would be appropriate at other times. This negotiation involved three parts (ego states), the rage part that threw his dog off the balcony, the wise part that would be given the role to decide how anger should be expressed, and the assertive part that would take on a larger role. All parts were able to agree on their new and revised roles.

4.5   *Panic Attacks*

Ego State Therapy is an excellent intervention for panic attack. One of two conditional situations, or a combination of the two, causes panic attacks. Panic attacks result from either an underlying ego state coming to the executive with unresolved severe trauma from a past phenomenon, or an underlying ego state coming to the executive that has consistently taken on the residuals from non-assertive expression. Panic attacks may also result from an interactive combination of these two causes. Each of the two situations may result in an ego state feeling overwhelmed and unable to cope, and when this ego state comes to the executive a severe loss of control is experienced. The following two sections will further define the two situational causes of panic attacks.

4.5.1   *Panic Attacks Stemming from Unresolved Trauma*

A traumatic experience that has been processed will not result in panic attacks. If a child, or an adult, is able to talk about the trauma that was experienced and feel closure with the incident, it will not continue to cause active problems in later life. It is the unresolved traumas that can become problematic.

There is an aspect of the way we learn that demands us to understand, and finish what is not understood. This trait serves us well, supplying energy to continue working on a problem until there is a completion. When someone asked you the name of someone who you know, but you just can't think of the name, you may feel frustrated until the name is yours. Before you think of the name, anything that reminds you that you have not remembered it will bring back that frustration. When we live through a, sometimes life threatening, trauma that was filled with frightening and severe affect, until we can feel closure with that trauma, reminders of it will bring back that severe affect. When the affect was one of being frightened and out of control, reminders of it will cause a panic attack with those same feelings. An example will better illustrate this.

Laura reported experiencing panic attacks when she was in a crowded place with people pressing against her (Emmerson, Video Tape, 1999). She reported experiencing a difficulty in breathing and a tightness around the throat, and having a need to rip something away from her neck. She experienced a fear of dying and a desperate need to get away from those pressing against her.

The Resistance Bridge Technique (section 2.2.4) was used to locate the traumatized ego state that was associated with the panic attack. Moving from the feelings of the panic attack to the first occurrence of those feelings, a ten-year-old little girl ego state emerged in severe distress. Questioning revealed she was caught in an ocean rip tide being kept from the beach. She could not touch the bottom and her little cousin was on her back, choking her; he, himself trying to keep from drowning. She thought she was going to die. She was able to make it back to the beach, and after being saved she was too frightened to tell her parents of the incident. She carried the unprocessed trauma with her, hiding it from her parents, and when she experienced being crowded and unable to move, that trauma returned, complete with the severe anxiety of the original incident. Before the ego state hypnotic session she was unaware of the connection between the panic attacks and the near drowning incident. The following is a transcript of selected parts of the therapy session. The transcript begins after a hypnotic induction:

> **Therapist**: Are you aware of that feeling you talked about earlier around the throat?
>
> **Client:** *(nods and verbalizes)* Yes.
>
> **Therapist**: What does that feel like for you?
>
> **Client:** Tightness.
>
> **Therapist**: Tightness. Just tell me exactly what you are experiencing now.
>
> **Client:** Movement around my eyes.
>
> **Therapist**: Um Hmm. That's interesting, isn't it? And what else?
>
> **Client:** Color, blue, but black *(starts crying)*.

Therapist: How do you feel about that blue, but black? Any feelings, or not?

Client: Polarity. A sense of calm, but also apprehension.

Therapist: Tell me about that sense of apprehension. *(pause)* That's right. Have the courage to go into that a bit and explore it a bit and report back.

Client: It's very dark and I'm afraid.

Therapist: Uh Hmm. It's very dark and you are afraid. *(Client crying more)* How old do you feel when you are feeling that very dark and afraid feeling?

Client: *(still crying)* Ten maybe.

Therapist: Ten. I would like for you to go to when you are ten years old feeling that same feeling. Are you inside or outside?

Client: *(crying)* Outside.

Therapist: Are you alone or with someone else?

Client: *(crying deeply)* I'm with people.

Therapist: It's OK I'm right here with you. I'm not going to leave you. Tell me what's happened?

Client: *(crying more loudly)* I'm in the water.

Therapist: Are you in the water?

Client: *(nods yes)* I'm in the water. *(Words are coming out through lots of tears)*.

Therapist: Yeah. That's OK. I'm right here with you. What's happening? *(pause with more crying)* I'm right here with you.

Client: *(having trouble getting her breath through the tears)* I can't swim.

Therapist: I can understand. That is really scary. Who else is with you there?

Client: I have my sister with me and some *(tears)* cousins.

Therapist: Uh Hmm. Do they know you are afraid?

Client: *(very distressed)* They're all. We can't swim. We are caught in a rip. We are being taken out to sea.

Therapist: Oh. That's very, very scary. I'm right here with you. Nothing is going to happen because I am right here with you. I'm not going to let anything happen.

Client: And my little cousin is littler than me, and he is climbing onto my shoulders *(loud crying and expression of fear)*.

Therapist: I see. I see. He is climbing onto your shoulders. And, and tell me what the outcome to this is. What happens in the end?

Client: *(much more calm)* Somebody saves us.

Therapist: So everybody gets saved?

Client: Uh. Hmm.

Therapist: OK. So lets go back to that rip. And your little cousin is climbing onto your shoulders. What would you like to say to your little cousin?

Client: He can't help it. He's little.

Therapist: He can't help it. You don't want to send him away, do you? Because he is little.

Client: *(shakes her head no)*

Therapist: But your afraid, aren't you?

Client: *(nods yes)*

Therapist: Is there anyone there you can ask for help?

Client: *(crying)* There's nobody around, because they don't know that we are there.

Therapist: OK. We are going to change this seen. Because you're afraid because you don't have anything to hang onto, aren't you?

Client: *(Nods)*

Therapist: OK. We can change this, because this is something you are carrying around with you. This isn't reality now. It actually happened, but you are carrying this with you. And we are going to give you a nice life preserver; a really strong one. And your cousin can hang onto your back and it wont make you sink.

Client: *(tears drying, speaking calmly)* There is somebody there.

Therapist: OK. Who is there now?

Client: An angel.

Therapist: An angel.

Client: *(Nods yes)*

Therapist: Uh. Huh. Tell me what's happening.

Client: *(calmly)* They say it's OK. I can breath. It doesn't matter.

Therapist: Oh. That's nice. It makes you feel much more calm, doesn't it?

Client: Uh Hmm.

Therapist: Uh Hmm. What can you say to that angel?

Client: *(deep breath)* I'll die.

Therapist: And what does the angel say to you?

Client: It doesn't matter.

Therapist: I want to tell you a secret. What can I call you, when you are ten years old there?

Client: Frightened.

Therapist: Frightened?

Client: Uh Hmm.

Therapist: Frightened, I want to tell you a secret. You, you are frightened. I understand that, and you fear you are going to die, but the secret is, you are not going to die. You are going to live. You are going to come through this, and I would like you to become less frightened, right there where you are. I'm going to give you a life preserver that you can hang onto, right from the very beginning. A really solid, secure life preserver. Can you feel it? It is right there in front of you.

(Child ego states love secrets and generally respond very well to them. It is a way of enhancing their attention to what is begin said.)

Client: *(nods yes, and whispers)* OK.

143

Therapist: OK. And frightened, I'm going to do something else. I am going to get another part to come in and help make you feel better. OK?

Client: *(whispers)* OK.

Therapist: OK. We really want you to feel better. OK. Thank you 'frightened' for talking with me. I am going to want to talk with you more in a minute, but I want to talk to, possibly an older state or a state that is mature and is wanting and able to help 'frightened' be less frighten. To protect 'frightened', and be there with 'frightened' there in the water with that life preserver, and help her feel more secure and safe. I would like for that part to come forward and speak with me now when it is ready to talk. Just say, I'm here. *(pause)* A state that likes to protect. Likes to nurture.

Client: Only the guardian angel.

Therapist: Only the guardian angel.

Client: *(Nods yes)*.

Therapist: Is the guardian angel part of you or is that separate from you?

Client: It's a part of me.

Therapist: OK. May I speak with the guardian angel please?

Client: *(Nods yes) (speaking very calmly)* I'm here.

Therapist: Guardian angel. Thank you for talking with me. You're aware about frightened, aren't you?

Client: Uh Hmm.

Therapist: Would you like to go and help frightened not be so 'frightened'?

Client: *(Nods yes)* Uh Hmm.

Therapist: Is it OK if 'frightened' has you and hangs onto the life preserver at the same time? And she can help her little cousin and feel good about it?

Client: *(nods yes)*

Therapist: I appreciate that frightened. And maybe when you go to, I mean 'guardian angel' I appreciate that, and maybe when you go to 'frightened' you can put your arm around her and help hold her too and make her feel better. Make sure that she knows she is not going to sink. Is that OK with you 'guardian angel'?

Client: Um hmm.

Therapist: I appreciate your help. Anything you want to tell me about yourself, 'guardian angel'?

Client: I was there with her all along.

Therapist: Yeah. And I think you probably helped her at the time. And now you can help her even more, uh, feel better about it, and resolved about it. OK?

Client: *(Nods yes)*.

Therapist: OK, lets go to 'frightened' now and put your arm around her and make her feel snug and that she's held up, and that she is not going to sink, and we know that she is not going to sink. And you can both feel the life preserver. And, 'Frightened', are you there. Can you feel the 'guardian angel'?

Client: *(Smiles broadly and calmly, nods yes)*

Therapist: How do you feel now 'frightened'?

Client: Feels safe.

Therapist: Everything is going to be OK, isn't it?

Client: *(Quickly and strongly nods yes)* Um Hmm.

Therapist: And 'frightened' can you feel your little cousin and you know you are going to save him.

Client: *(searching expression)*

Therapist: On your back?

Client: No.

Therapist: Doesn't matter. It doesn't matter.

Client: I don't know what happened to him.

Therapist: But he, we know he's OK.

Client: *(quick nod yes)* Um Hmm. *(calm and happy)*

Therapist: Any other feelings there that need to be resolved, 'frightened'?

Client: *(head goes down, and nods yes)*

Therapist: Tell me about those 'frightened'. I'm here to listen.

Client: *(starts crying and rubbing eyes)*

Therapist: What is it?

Client: *(through tears)* I can't tell my mum and dad.

Therapist: Pardon me?

Client: I can't tell my mum and dad.

Therapist: You're embarrassed?

Client: I'll get into trouble.

Therapist: I see. I see. Did you know? *(I decided to phrase the question in a more open fashion)* Do you think your mum and dad love you, Frightened?

Client: Sometimes.

Therapist: Uh huh. What would you like to tell them?

Client: That I was really frightened.

Therapist: Um hmm. Lets, I would like to go with you to your mum and dad now and

Client: *(crying loudly)* I don't want to go.

Therapist: OK. OK. Would you like me to tell your mum and dad?

Client: I still might get into trouble.

Therapist: Well, let me tell you something Frightened. I will guarantee you, ah, with what we do here you're not going to get into trouble. Can you hear my voice. I can guarantee you that you are not going to get into trouble because we are going to make sure that your mum and dad understand. And even if they, even if they were frightened we are going to understand their feelings.

Client: OK.

Therapist: OK, lets go to your mum and dad. Do you want me to tell them first or do you want to tell them?

Client: You tell them.

Therapist: OK. Can you see your mum and dad there?

Client: Um Hmm.

Therapist: What can I call them?

Client: Mum and Dad.

Therapist: OK, Mum and Dad, I've got something to tell you about your little girl. She had a really frightening experience, and she has been helped allot, ah, and see feels better about that experience, but she is real nervous about you, because she knows that at some level that you love her and she's afraid you are going to be upset with her. She is afraid you are going to be upset with her, and it is really scary to her. And what she really needs to hear is how you love her and how happy you are that she is OK.

Client: *(stops crying)*

Therapist: What are they doing 'frightened'?

Client: Hugging me.

Therapist: Huh! How does that feel?

Client: *(moves shoulders like she is being hugged)* Feels good.

Therapist: That's fantastic, isn't it?

Client: *(Nods yes)*

Therapist: What can you say to them?

Client: *(shifts shoulders up and down)* I don't know?

Therapist: Do you love them?

Client: Um Hmm.

Therapist: Do you want to tell them?

Client: *(nods yes)*

Therapist: What do they say?

Client: They say that they love me too, and that I should always know that I can go and tell them things.

147

Therapist: That's nice, isn't it?

Client: *(Nods yes)*

Therapist: Can, ah, can you give them a hug too?

Client: *(quick and happy smile, nods yes)*

Therapist: That's fantastic. Do you still want to be called frightened or do you want to be called something else?

Client: *(Loudly and proudly)* Brave.

Therapist: Brave! That's fantastic, isn't it?

Client: *(Nods yes, smiling)*

Therapist: OK 'Brave', I want to ask you a question? In the past when this person has had those panic attacks, was that associated with 'frightened'?

Client: Um Hmm.

Therapist: And now you feel brave!

Client: *(Big yes nods)*

Therapist: And you know that you can handle things and guardian angel is going to be there, and you know that Mummy and Daddy love you.

Client: *(Big yes nod)*

Therapist: That's fantastic, isn't it?

Client: Um Hmm.

It was important to empower the state that had the fearful experience and had held onto the fear of drowning, so it would no longer had the need to carry that fear, and to help the little girl state to feel a completion by talking with her parents. With that resolution of both fears, the fear of drowning and the fear of telling the parents, Laura was able to experience a completion, a resolution. Like you, when you finally remember the name you have been trying to think of, and thereafter you are not bothered by something that reminds you of that person, she was able to be in a crowded situation without distress.

4.5.2 Panic Attacks Stemming from Residuals of Non-Assertive Behavior

It is often the case that individuals who experience panic attacks present as very nice people, people who rarely demonstrate anger, or even with an affect of being slightly upset. They are often considered to be very easy to get along with. If fact, they may be too easy to get along with for their own best mental health. By denying others of hearing their true feelings, they also deny themselves a venting of those feelings.

It is impossible to interact with people without frustrations and angers sometimes resulting. These frustrations and angers need to be expressed an appropriate ways. We need to feel expressed, and when we feel unable to express we may feel "bottled up". This is an accurate feeling in relation to what is happening with our ego states. These frustrations and angers are often held by a covert state that rarely comes to the executive. It takes on these negative emotions, feeling more and more weighed down by them. If they are not released the build-up will eventually become too exaggerated, and the covert state that holds them will come to the executive. Often this is an internal state that does not know how to deal with being executive. The combination of the heavy build-up of frustration and anger, and the covert state being forced to the executive results in a feeling of severe anxiety and a feeling of being out of control.

Treatment of this type of panic attack is dependent upon the client learning better internal communication, and a better usage of ego states. It is important that the ego state that takes on the frustration and anger learn to work with an ego state that can be assertive so the negative feelings can be appropriately vented before the build-up becomes uncomfortable, and long before a panic attack results. The following is an example of this type of ego state resolution, also exerted from the Laura videotape:

Therapist: … I want to talk with another part that can teach people how to be assertive. That part is assertive itself, and it can teach people how to be assertive. *(Information about this part was gathered prior to hypnosis)*. Just say I'm here when you are ready to speak.

Client: *(Strongly)* I'm here.

Therapist: OK. What can I call you?

Client: Confident.

Therapist: Confident, thank you for talking with me, and Confident, I was talking with this person earlier and she said she is sometimes not very assertive with people she doesn't know very well, especially with men. I wonder if there is some way you could help her with this?

Client: Um Hmm, *(Nods head yes)* I can do that.

Therapist: I can see you are very confident.

Client: I am.

Therapist: And you have a lot of talents that could help her. Because when she, when she doesn't assert herself when she doesn't talk with men, that, ah, that causes her to take on things she doesn't need to carry around. And if you are assertive with, with the people she meets that could make her to feel really expressed and that she doesn't have to be burdened by carrying things around.

Client: Um Hmm.

Therapist: I would really appreciate that. Thank you Confident, and I want to talk with you again, but first I want to talk to a part that in the past hasn't been very assertive, has not been very assertive, especially if sometimes talking with men that she does not know very well. Just say, "I'm here" when you are here.

Client: *(quieter and more meekly)* I'm here.

Therapist: What can I call you?

Client: I don't know. The hidden one.

Therapist: Hidden one. Thank you for talking with me Hidden One. Did you hear what Confident said, that she is willing to help you, if you are willing to, to allow Confident to word with you?

Client: *(weakly)* Yeah, I heard.

Therapist: And, I get a sense that you are not too sure about that.

Client: Yeah.

Therapist: Can you tell me, can you tell me something that might help me to understand this?

Client: I didn't think that girls were allowed to be assertive.

Therapist: Um Hmm. Ah, what do you think now, hidden one?

Client: I don't think that they are allowed.

Therapist: They're not really allowed. When you are talking with me, even though you don't think they are allowed, can you, now I don't know the answer to this, but I would really like to hear it from you, can you give confident one permission to come out and help you out?

Client: *(very pleased)* She can do it if she wants.

Therapist: You're really happy with that, aren't you?

Client: *(smiling and nodding head, yes)*

Therapist: You're not too keen on sitting there and being nervous, are you?

Client: *(laughing)* She can do it!

Therapist: That's fantastic. Hey, I appreciate that hidden one, and I'm sure that you have things that you can do really well. You seem like a nice sensitive part and I am sure you have nice roles you can play.

Client: *(nods head, yes)*

Therapist: Is it OK if you tell Confident One now directly that she can she can help be assertive when you feel like it with men or with other people you don't know very well? *(pause)* What happened?

Client: *(smiling broadly)* She laughed. I said she can do it, I have no problems with that and she just laughed.

Therapist: OK. Thank you very much Hidden One. Confident, can I speak with you one more time please?

Client: *(head held higher)* Um Huh.

Therapist: Is that OK with you?

Client: *(laughing in good spirits)* Yes.

Therapist: That's OK with you too. It sounds like you and hidden one have really worked this out.

Client: *(nods head, yes)* Yes.

> **Therapist**: I appreciate that a lot. Before we stop are there any other states that, that I need to speak with?
>
> **Client:** No, we are all happy now.

This example demonstrates how ego state negotiation can help the client with internal communication where states can agree to take give up and take on situational roles. When states are happy with the re-balancing of roles, the changes tend to be permanent, and clients report real changes in the way they interact with the outside world. When panic attacks result from a state becoming burdened by continually taking on non-vented frustrations or anger it is important for a capable state to learn to work in the family of states in such a manner to appropriately vent these negative feelings.

4.5.3   Talking with a Person who is having a Panic Attack

An understanding of ego state theory in relation to panic attacks is useful in understanding techniques for helping a person out of panic, when they are not in therapy. This is a technique that non-therapists can use also, although it does not prevent the person from continuing to have panic attacks. Panic attacks, as discussed above, result from ego states that are feeling out of control becoming executive. Assisting the person into a different ego state, an ego state that feels in control, will result in the disappearance of the immediate panic symptoms. It is helpful to know the person in order to do this, but it is not essential.

If you know the person who is having a panic attack, you will know some of the person's ego states. Pick a state that the person often experiences and begin talking to that state, in order to bring it to the executive. For example, if the person is a grandmother and enjoys talking about a grandchild, Amy, start asking direct question about Amy. Be loud and clear in asking these Amy questions and do not respond to the panic state that is out. Just continue asking questions about Amy until the state that enjoys sharing information about Amy comes to the executive. Then continue talking about Amy until the person is well removed from the severe affect.

If you do not know the person who is having a panic attack you can begin taking loudly and directly to the person about something they can visually see. I once assisted a woman out of a panic attack by picking up a vase with a potted plant and started taking about the color and texture of the plant, and about how it could grow in that dirt. I asked direct questions, loudly and clearly about the plant and the pot. The woman begin to respond to my questions and after talking for a few moments about potted plants, and her experiences with them, she exhibited a relaxed and thoughtful state.

4.6 Ego State Therapy in the Treatment of Addictions

One of the most useful applications of Ego State Therapy is in the treatment of drug addiction and other addictions. Addictive behavior is often the result of negative feelings cause by one or more ego states. The addictive behavior may block the ego state and its associated negative feelings in such a way that it is difficult for the client to cease the behavior, because when the behavior is ceased the negative feelings return.

Various ego state configurations may contribute to addictive behavior. Ego State Therapy can result in resolving negative feelings associated with addictive behavior and in empowering ego states that have a clear understanding that the behavior is unwanted. Following a presentation of the use of Ego State Therapy to assist in healing a drug additive ego state structure, techniques will be presented for assisting clients in smoking cessation and controlling eating habits.

4.6.1 Drug Addiction

It is important to look at the relationship ego states have to drug addiction to understand how and when to best apply ego state techniques. Key to understanding this relationship is understanding that drugs can block ego states from being able to come to the executive. A particular drug can block one or more specific ego states from the executive and have little impact in blocking other states.

It is most usual that individuals who suffer from drug addictive behavior also suffer from traumatized ego states. When individuals speak of their 'drug of choice' they are often saying (without realizing it) that they have found a drug that is able to block a traumatized ego state that normally disrupts their lives. The drug of choice is the drug that allows relief from the experience of the traumatized ego state. The individual gains not only whatever positive experience the drug renders, but also relief from the trauma associated with the blocked state. This is a very appealing combination and many will return to it again and again. After a physical, or psychological dependency (or both), develops, in order to become clear of the dependency the individual has to deal with both breaking the dependency, and deal with the trauma of the reintroduced traumatized ego state.

Dr. John Lovern, speaking at the 1994 Milton H. Erickson Foundation spoke on the impact of drugs on states. (Dr. Lovern felt a large number of drug abusers were multiples with dissociative identity disorder. It is my view he was most often dealing with ego states, not alters. None-the-less, he enjoyed good success helping persons suffering from drug addiction, by attending to trauma held by underlying states.) The following is a quote from his presentation:

> You cannot treat dissociative identity disorder when they are using these heavy drugs that are drugging the system out, even if those heavy drugs that are drugging the system out are being dispensed by your friendly neighborhood psychiatrist. I've seen so many patients do poorly in therapy because you get to a certain point and you hit a wall because you have worked with the personalities that have an issue going and then you hit the ones that have the issue, but are asleep. So you have to get them off of that stuff. Dr. Lovern spoke concerning anti-depressants, "If it is just suppressing depressed parts then it is making them unavailable for psychotherapy, unavailable for change, and it is a temporary measure that is going to come apart later."

He spoke more generally of any psychoactive drugs, including illegal drug addiction and prescribed drugs:

> If you want to take over your personality system (if an ego state wants to take over) then one good way is take a drug that you are tolerant to and nobody else is. And take that continuously for a few years. Then you want to see chaos, take that person who you now know is addicted to that substance and take them off of it. They will have one hell of a withdrawal. First of all it is going to be a very hard withdrawal because they are addicted to something and there is a withdrawal syndrome that goes with it, but then all the disruptive personalities (states) that were sedated out of commission will wake up and raise heck. ... A drug can activate a state or it can inhibit a state. Or, it can activate a state by inhibiting another state that inhibits that state. ... You need to be alert in addiction or in medication of people in general with psychoactive substances in terms of what is being suppressed (what states are being suppressed), what (state) is being activated, what (state) is being accessed, which (state) is being sedated.

Bill Patterson is an ego state therapist who has enjoyed good success working with heroin attacks, both at a clinic in Melbourne, Australia (The clinic has a team of counselors, medical doctors and practitioners working in allied health fields), and in a separate private practice. The typical ego states he works with are states that are depressed, (he has not met an addict who has not experienced depression during addiction.), states that carry pain, fear, anger or sadness from trauma usually that occurred earlier in life, states with suicidal ideation, and states that manifest obsessive compulsive disorders. The following is a case study submitted by Bill Patterson of one of the addicts he has worked with at the clinic:

CASE STUDY—DARREN (pseudonym)

Two years ago, I was introduced to Darren by his Mother. He had been addicted to heroin for two years and was three months into a methadone maintenance program, as prescribed by his family doctor. Darren was 23 years of age, living at home with his mother and new partner, a younger brother and two sisters. His mother explained her concern with his reclusive behavior and long periods of time that Darren spent in his bedroom. She was also fearful that the methadone program might not be sufficient and that a relapse into heroin usage might occur.

Having mutually agreed that hypnosis might help this situation Darren underwent a total of eight sessions that utilized Ego State Therapy as the primary approach to the problems described. The first session was used to gain some information about Darren, establish a bond of trust, and to explore Darren's capacity to bring out states through some preliminary experiences in trance. He told me of his life over the past few years. His older brother, unemployed, had left the family home for the street scene and had developed a heroin habit. Darren was strongly supportive of his brother, and due to his brother's connections, Darren started to use heroin and developed an addiction. He soon abandoned his established friends whom he felt were not approving and tended then to keep to himself, spending many hours each day locked away in his room.

Because of his addiction, he explained he had lost his confidence and desire to socialize with the family or any others. He felt that hypnosis might offer a way to help him change his current lack of mental "well being". He expressed a strong desire to make changes as he could remember times when he was happy. Darren felt it would be good to reduce his dependence on methadone, to stay clean from heroin, and in general to get a boost in confidence. He also wanted to find a girlfriend as his previous girlfriend had left, principally due to the addiction.

We then agreed it might be interesting to experience what it could be like to go into hypnosis. It is usually quite easy to elicit "parts" or states with just a light hypnotic state and Darren was able to do this in the first session, with little explanation of the process of how our mood or personality states comprise a whole unified self.

A number of parts were identified in the first session that subsequently reappeared in further sessions including:

- "Moby", who kept him thinking all the time and was responsible for his insomnia.
- "Darro", who liked to joke and have fun and "helped him get by".

- "Paul", the part that was addicted and did not have to do anything.
- "Shand", a good adviser but quite serious and did not approve of Darro.
- "Dave", a reclusive part that was sad and felt alone.
- "Peter", a shy and younger state.

(Ego states most often give themselves a name that defines their role, although it is not unusual for them to give Christian names.) 'Moby' was the first part that appeared in response to the question:

Therapist: If there is a part that can tell me about Darren's addiction, just say I'm here?

Darren: I'm here.

Therapist: Thanks for speaking with me, is there a name I can call you?

Darren: Yeah...call me Moby.

Therapist: What do you do for Darren, Moby?

Darren: Well, I keep him up all night.

Therapist: How do you do that?

Darren: By making him think.

Therapist: By making him think?

Darren: Yeah...I keep him thinking. He has to think.

Therapist: How long have you been with him, Moby?

Darren: Four years, since starting *(referring to smoking marijuana then eventually injecting heroin)*.

Therapist: And you keep him thinking, so he stays up at night a lot? *(Darren's concern with his insomnia.)*

Darren: Yeah...I keep him thinking all night. He needs to think a lot about what he is doing.

Therapist: Is there a part that you know about, that makes your job more difficult?

157

Darren: Yeah…there is a part that doesn't like me.

Therapist: Thanks for talking with me, Moby. I appreciate it and would like to talk with you again perhaps if that's alright…I would like to talk to the part that Moby spoke about.

Darren: Yes. *(Darren's voice tone and facial expression changed to reflect lightness and humor.)*

Therapist: What name can I call you, part.

Darren: Darro.

Therapist: What role do you play for Darren?

Darren: I help him get by. I keep him laughing. If he didn't have me it would be real bad.

Therapist: Real bad?

Darren: I help him keep his head.

Therapist: So you give him his sense of humor, Darro?

Darren: Sometimes…I don't do it as much now since Moby became so big.

Therapist: Oh yes? Can you tell me why that is?

Darren: Because he has lost something. He doesn't want me when *that* part is there.

Therapist: Tell me about that part, I would really like to know about that part.

Darren: That part is always around.

Therapist: Would it be all right to talk to that part and if it is listening could you let me know?

Darren: Yeah…*(slow talking, quiet voiced part speaking)* I'm here.

Therapist: Is there a name I can call you?

Darren: Paul.

Therapist: What is it you do for Darren, Paul?

Darren: I help him cope with things.

Therapist: You help him cope with things?

Darren: Yeah…so he doesn't have to do anything.

Therapist: How do you do that…help so he doesn't have to do things.

Darren: I let him know what it is like when he has a hit, when he needs *the feeling.*

Therapist: How long have you been with him?

Darren: Four years.

Therapist: Four years, do you know Moby? He's been with him since four years ago as well?

Darren: Yeah, Moby and I get on well. Moby helps me. We keep him from feeling too much and when he needs to get away from everyone. Moby keeps him thinking and I help him to cope.

Therapist: Do you know Darro?

Darren: I know Darro. He doesn't like me at all. I stop him from laughing and having fun. Darro really hates me and he is a lot smaller now.

As the session continued more information was gained about the communication and relationship between "Paul" who was connected with the need to take drugs and "Moby", the part that produced the insomnia. Both parts were in conflict with "Darro", the part of Darren that liked to have fun and helped him get by. As the dialogue brought more insight into relationship dynamics another part was identified in the role of good adviser. This good adviser, "Shand", seemed rather serious and declared his purpose was to help Darren keep up with tasks that needed to be done such as self grooming, cleaning, cutting hair, and so on.

When asked if he could help Darren by giving him advise on how he might sleep better and to slow down the thinking, Shand said he would try but didn't feel strong enough. The session was concluded by ego strengthening suggestions for Shand and agreement that we would look at some ways of helping Darren in a future session. At the end of this session Darren reported feeling lighter and seemed to be more optimistic about his situation expressing surprise at how his parts seemed to have a mind of their own.

The next week Darren arrived and entered into a trance quite easily. During this session a shy ego state, "Peter", surfaced. This state helped Darren to be quiet and remain unnoticed. This part told me that he helped Darren get through life, but was shy and didn't want him to stand out. He seemed somewhat distressed and I asked the part to tell me how old it felt, as that feeling became more intense. Through this affect bridge he regressed to an experience when, at five years of age, he recalled sitting in the back of a classroom with the teacher asking him a question. He was unable to answer as he did not understand the letters on the board (he later told me that he had experienced considerable learning difficulties) and the teacher made humiliating remarks that left him feeling embarrassed and ashamed.

At this point Darren's emotional level of expression suddenly increased into a full-scale abreaction. This memory was followed by two other similar experiences where Darren was 16-years-old and in technical college and 19-years-old where he was attending an adult educational program. In both these instances he was asked a question that he was unable to answer and suffered extreme self-consciousness that led to a profound sense of shame. In each situation he felt diminished in the eyes of his peers. As he reviewed these memories as an "adult" part he realized he saw himself as significantly inferior to others and felt he had none of the necessary basic skills that one gains from school. As we explored these ideas we discovered some skills that Darren did in fact possess which included an ability to socialize and therefore network with others.

He became aware, through metaphor, that many people in life became successful and were held in high esteem, yet their academic levels were only modest. Darren was able to develop an insight into a feeling of inadequacy that had been internalized and maintained most of his life. He felt the influence of this feeling on his addiction was significant and he was able to refocus and work towards more life-fulfilling self concepts through visualizing himself in successful situations. 'Dave' and 'Peter' were parts that had a close relationship and were responsible for Darren feeling shy and alone. These parts help Darren visualize demonstrating social skills and feeling the positive responses from others.

During several further sessions, previous ego states were elicited and other issues that were connected to the separation of Darren's father and mother were addressed and processed. Agreements were reached with Paul (addiction), Moby (insomnia), and Shand (a helpful adviser) to help Darren develop his new skills, and to do this he will need energy to interact more with others and that he could do this by starting to leave his bedroom more often. He would start by joining the family for meals and contacting old friends (pre drug use). He could develop his skills. Further sessions reinforced this insight and brought about agreements with the other states to change some of the old ways for new, interesting and creative ways of doing things.

Darren's mother informed me some weeks after the last session that there had been some pleasing changes. Darren had continued no use of heroin, was reducing his dosage of methadone and was joining in with the family. He was regaining some of his old sense of humor and fun, he had renewed some friendships from some years past, and he seemed more confident.

More recent news was that Darren is happily involved in a relationship and is remaining clean of heroin.

SUMMARY
An important aspect from the case study above is the work that was completed to resolve past traumas so they would no longer interfere with the changes Darren wanted for his life. Ego states carrying trauma can be blocked by specific drugs and the combination of the positive feelings gained from these drugs with the additional relief from the underlying feelings of trauma can make drug addictive behavior difficult to resist. Individuals who have resolved traumatic issues will have a greater ability to avoid addictive behavior.

Once an individual has a physical drug addiction, the difficulty in dealing with the physical withdrawals and at the same time dealing with the reawakening of ego states that hold trauma can make it extremely difficult to become free from the 'drug of choice'. This difficulty is exacerbated by the manner non-blocked ego states have become accustomed to the absence of the drug blocked states.

Ego State Therapy for the resolution of trauma can not only make it less likely that an individual would yield to drug addition, but it can assist the person attempting to break an addiction by resolving the traumatized states and assisting all states to rebalance roles, following the cessation of the drug usage. It is important to remember that Ego State Therapy cannot resolve childhood trauma of states while those states are being blocked by a psychoactive substance.

4.6.2 *Smoking Cessation and Diet Control*

Hypnosis is often viewed as a good tool to assist clients who want to quit smoking, or clients who want to change the amount or type of food they consume. It has often been used with techniques using direct suggestion relating to the smoking or eating. A problem with this approach is that if the addictive behavior is present to help block the unwanted feelings stemming underlying trauma, the suggestions will be only a temporary solution. The negative energy from the underlying trauma will often cause the return of the addictive behavior.

The ego state intervention that is presented here is the same for either smoking cessation or diet control. It locates and resolves any trauma that the behavior may be masking and empowers states that want healthier behavior.

Some cautions relating to diet control should first be noted. There is a great deal of social pressure associated with a thin body. A client should not be helped to lose weight if he or she is already under a healthy weight. This client may be suffering from an eating disorder and it is the disorder that needs to be addressed, not weight loss. There are also clients who are the same weight as other members of their families of the same gender when they were the same age. These clients may already be at their set point weight and attempting to maintain a lower weight may feel like a starvation diet. Their weight may have nothing to do with dysfunctional ego states, and self-esteem issues may be a better focus in counseling. It is good to discuss with these clients about the occasions they eat more than they would like in order to determine if hunger is the cause of this eating, or if some sort of stress, anxiety, or trance-like state seems to be associated with their eating. It is unethical for a therapist to assist a client to an unhealthy weight.

Smoking or unhealthy eating may be merely habit related and not related to any underlying trauma. If this is the case ego state negotiation techniques are the most useful intervention. It is preferred to determine if a trauma is associated with the unwanted behavior, if it is, to resolve the trauma, and if not to proceed with ego state negotiation techniques. The following steps include trauma resolution. If it is determined in steps seven and eight that a trauma is not associated with the unwanted behavior proceed to step 10 and continue with ego state negotiation techniques.

The ego state intervention for smoking or diet control will be presented in point form then each point will be discussed. It is assumed in using this technique that the above cautions have been taken into account:

1. Discuss with the client the nature of the addictive behavior.
2. Find out when the client is most likely to succumb to addictive behavior?
3. Get a detailed account of a particular instance of addictive behavior.
4. Ask the client to explain why the addictive behavior is not wanted.
5. Hypnotize the client.
6. Use information gained from step 3 above to take the client to the time when addictive behavior occurred and focus on the anxiety associated with needing the behavior.
7. Increase the affect of the anxiety until the client exhibits clear emotion.
8. Use the affect bridge to discover the unresolved issues associated with the addictive behavior.

9. Use techniques described in the Tools for Processing Trauma section (3.1.4) to resolve associated issues and empower the associated ego state.
10. Ask to speak with the part of the person that knows it does not want the addiction; the part that was speaking in step 3 above.
11. Get a name for that part that knows it does not want the addiction (see General Guidelines for Talking with Ego States, section 2.2.2).
12. Negotiate with that part that does not want the behavior to come to the executive at those times when addictive behavior has previously occurred (from step 2 above).
13. Using imagery, place the client in scenes when previously addictive behavior might have occurred and ask the client to see how temptation is managed.
14. If temptation is managed well bring the client out of hypnosis, otherwise determine what extra ego state work needs to be finished before ending the hypnosis session.
15. Debrief with the client describing the ego state dynamics that have been used to resolve trauma and empower that ego state.

Each step will now be discussed.

1. *Discuss with the client the nature of the addictive behavior.*
   Whether the client wants to focus on smoking, eating, or some other additive behavior it is important to gather information relating to the behavior. How long has the unwanted behavior been practiced? What is the extent of practice? Was anything memorable happening in the life of the client when the behavior began? What is currently associated with the behavior? For example, nervousness, stress, feeling out of control, feeling social pressure, etc. Why does the client want to stop the behavior?

2. *Find out when the client is most likely to succumb to addictive behavior?*
   It is important to gather information concerning the times the client has been vulnerable to the unwanted behavior. If smoking is the unwanted behavior, those times might be during a coffee, with friends during a break at work, after breakfast, or at a nightclub. If the unwanted behavior is eating more than desired, the vulnerable times might be when arriving home

from work, after satiation, during boredom, or when upset. Record in detail the information gathered, as it will be needed in later steps.

3. *Get a detailed account of a particular instance of addictive behavior.* This information will later be used to help the hypnotized client to bring to the executive the ego state that practices the unwanted behavior. Ask the client questions that will allow you later to build the scene where the behavior was practiced. Gather sensory information, such as a visual description of the room, where the light comes from, the texture of a couch or table, the temperature, feelings, physical sensations, sense of control, if other people present, etc.

4. *Ask the client to explain why the addictive behavior is not wanted.* The first three steps gives you the information required to have the needed understanding of the addiction, and to assist the client into the addicted ego state, once hypnotized. Step four allows an ego state that does not want the behavior to give expression. Notes should be taken concerning why the client does not want the behavior so at the appropriate time they can be repeated and used to bring to the executive a state that does not want the addiction. This state will be taught to take the executive during times when the client has been most susceptible to the addiction in the past.

5. *Hypnotize the client.* Use the technique you prefer to hypnotize the client. A hypnotic depth of medium to deep is preferred, although a light/ medium state can used.

6. *Use information gained from step 3 above to take the client to the time when addictive behavior occurred and focus on the anxiety associated with needing the behavior.* This anxiety can be boredom, a need to relax, a feeling of social pressure, or any feeling that precedes the behavior. Ask the client to have the courage to really go into that feeling, and when this question is asked make sure to repeat the feeling in the client's own words. For example, if the client has said that a feeling of "Nothing really matters" is being experienced a statement such as the following could be made: "A feeling that

nothing really matters; I would like you to have the courage to really experience that feeling that nothing really matters. Go inside it and tell me more about exactly how that feels."

7.   *Increase the affect of the anxiety until the client exhibits clear emotion.*
     As the client is clearly and overtly experiencing the feeling (not talking about it from outside the feeling, but telling about it from the experience), ask the client on a scale of 1 to 100 how much is "Nothing really matters" being experienced presently? If the client says 60 and there is little or no affect being overtly exhibited, ask the client, "I wonder if you can get that up to 70?" Continue to urge the client to increase the feeling until a clear overt affect is exhibited. If after several efforts to determine if an anxiety is associated with the unwanted behavior the client reports no anxiety, proceed to step 10 with ego state negotiation techniques.

8.   *Use the affect bridge to discover the unresolved issues associated with the addictive behavior.*
     When the client exhibits clear affect asked, "Feeling those feelings (repeat them in the clients own words) as you are right now, how old do you feel? Go to when you were (name the age the client has given you) right now, when you experienced (repeat feelings) for the first time." For example, "Go to when you were about seven, first experiencing really feeling that nothing really matters." Use affect in you voice to match the affect of the client. Then continuing with the affect in your voice ask, "Are you inside or outside?" Given an answer ask, "Are you alone or with someone else?" Given an answer say, "Tell me exactly what is happening." These questions may need to be varied, due to the depth of the hypnosis or the nature of the client. Make sure to continue to respond to the specific client and keep the direction moving to the first experience of the feelings, the same feelings that the client experiences when addictive behavior occurs.

9.   *Use techniques described in the Tools for Processing Trauma section (3.1.4) to resolve associated issues and empower the associated ego state.*
     Make sure:

1. that the client expresses, overcoming fear,

2. that the fear producing agent is removed or changed, and

3. that the state that had held the unresolved feelings get all needs met (see section 3.1.4 for the detail needed to resolve trauma). It is important that all this occur while the client is in the state that first experienced the negative feelings that are related to the addictive behavior.

10. *Ask to speak with the part of the person that knows it does not want the addiction; the part that was speaking in step 3 above.*
    Use the information gathered in step three to bring out the ego state that really does not want the person to continue with the additive behavior. A good way to do this is to repeat much of what the client said about that part in the client's own words. For example, "Now I want to talk with that part of you that really does not want to smoke, the part that does not like the bad breath, that is concerned about health problems and smoking."

11. *Get a name for that part that knows it does not want the addiction (see General Guidelines for Talking with Ego States, section 2.2.2).*
    After beginning a conversation with the part that does not want the addiction to continue, ask it, "What can I call this part of you that knows it does not want to continue eating between meals?" It is important to get a name so you can quickly and easily call that part back again without having to define it with several sentences. If it has difficulty giving a name for itself you can suggest one, "Would 'Health Conscious' be a good name for you?"

12. *Negotiate with that part that does not want the behavior, to come to the executive at those times when addictive behavior has previously occurred (from step 2 above).*
    At this point you have some very useful information. You know when the addictive behavior normally is problematic and you know a state that does not want the addictive behavior to occur. If the state that is against the addictive behavior can come to the executive during times of temptation the person will not give in to the behavior. This sounds simple. Just bring to the executive a state that does not want the behavior and the behavior disappears. The problem is that the state that

wants the behavior will often jump into the executive during times of temptation. Therefore, negotiation between the state that wants the behavior and the state that does not want the behavior needs to result in an agreement that both can feel positive toward. It may be helpful to bring in other states for such an agreement to be successful. For example, if a client smokes during times when insecurity is felt, a third state (secure state) may agree to help the insecure state so it can give permission for the non-addictive state to come to the executive.

13. *Using imagery, place the client in scenes when previously addictive behavior might have occurred and ask the client to see how tempta-tion is managed.*

    When it appears that a negotiation has resulted in the states being balanced in such a way that the non-addictive state will be free to assume the executive during times of temptation, imagery can be used to check the new alignment of states. This accomplishes two things. It allows the therapist and the client to see if the ego state work has been successful in making it easier for the client to control the addiction, and it gives the client confidence that success over the addiction is within his or her control.

14. *If temptation is managed well bring the client out of hypnosis, oth-erwise determine what extra ego state work needs to be finished before ending the hypnosis session.*

    It may be necessary to carry out more ego state negotiation before the client can feel secure. Occasionally, even though one trauma has been resolved, a different trauma needs resolution, and this can be determined when temptation imagery is used test the success of the session. Continue with any additional ego state work, according to need, until, when the temptation imagery is used, the client feels secure about avoiding the additive behavior.

15. *Debrief with the client describing the ego state dynamics that have been used to resolve trauma and empower that ego state.*

    It is a good practice to share with the client any information that gives a better understanding of how the work will be helpful. Clients who feel informed about the process are more likely to feel empowered. This feeling of being part of the process is especially helpful to clients who are seeking more control in their lives.

4.7   Multiple Personality (Dissociative Identity Disorder)

This section describes some important aspects of working with clients who have dissociative identity disorder. Working with multiples is one of the most difficult and demanding tasks a therapist can take on, and this work requires a highly trained and skilled therapist. Ego state theory and practice can enhance work with multiples and it is a valuable tool for this work, but this book should not be considered sufficient training for this type of work.

Dissociative identity disorder may be the result of chronic and severe child abuse. The normal ego state structure is disturbed by a need to escape the pain of abuse. Over months (usually years) of severe abuse certain children learn to 'not remember' the abuse when they change ego states. For example, during school the next day, they may not recall what happened the night before. The communication between surface ego states is broken down, for the coping of the child.

While the non-multiple person will be able to have a relatively clear memory of what happened while in a different surface ego state, the multiple may not be able to recall what occurred just a few seconds before, due to stitching alters (the separated ego states of multiples). A non-multiple may go to the fridge, open it, and think, "Now, why did I come in here?" The multiple may open the fridge and think, "How did I get home, and how long have I been here?" A multiple will experience blackouts during the day from which memories are not accessible. During the time of the blackout a different alter was out and the next time that alter becomes executive the memories of its past are available. If a multiple is asked, "Were you ever abused as a child?" the answer is usually an honest, "No". The alter that is answering has no memories of being abused. Great detail of the abuse can be given when talking with the alter that was abused.

The therapist should be careful to clarify to states that there is no goal to get rid of a state when working with ego states. States will

169

not cooperate if they believe you want to get rid of them. This is especially true when working with alters. Many multiples have states that fear a therapist would try to cease their existence. It often takes months, sometimes years, of work for the different alters to feel comfortable enough to talk and come to the executive. This process is slowed if some of the states fear for their existence. The following are some reasons alters are reluctant to speak, or find it difficult to speak:

- They may fear the therapist will try to get rid of them.
- They may fear the therapist will keep them from doing what they believe they must do.
- They may often not be able to hear the therapist.
- They may prefer to keep trauma hidden.

It is not unusual for an alter to believe the person will die if it does not do its job. Even if the role of an alter is to be hard and mean, it can believe that it has to be this way or great pain will come to the person. This may have been the case at some point in the past, during the chronic abuse. A hard, mean state may have helped protect the person. In adulthood the hard, mean state may bring much distress to the person. Ego state negotiation can result in a malevolent alter agreeing to take on a more positive role.

Communication between alters is very poor. Some alters will be able to communicate with each other, and it is possible for a multiple to have surface alters that have recall from when a different alter was executive, recall like we have with ego states. Some alters exhibit practically no communication with each other, even other surface alters. Because communication between alters is so poor, often many alters cannot hear what the therapist is saying. New alters may appear after months of work, and report no recognition of what has been said in therapy. It is the goal of ego state work with multiples to assist alters into roles that can be acceptable to every alter and to increase communication between alters. Alters may be introduced to each other and convinced to continue to communicate so memories can be shared. They must learn to trust each other to make this possible.

A further goal for working with multiples is to process the trauma that is held. This can be a difficult task, and it can take much quality work even to get to the state(s) that hold the trauma. The coping style of the multiple has been to bury and hide trauma; trauma that has been so difficult that the person could cope in no other way than to believe it did not happen. Understanding and resolution are foreign concepts for these traumatized, isolated states, and often for alters that have learned to protect the person by keeping the trauma hidden. These traumatized states are non-accustomed to being helped, or to feeling better.

Ego state techniques to resolve trauma and to improve internal communication can bring relief and re-integration to a person with dissociative identity disorder. It is not the goal of the therapy to make a single personality, but to make an integrated personality with resolved, respecting states, much like the ego states of the non-clinical population.

4.8 *Post Traumatic Stress Disorder (PTSD)*

The symptoms of PTSD have become well known, and few would dispute that some clients react pathologically due to previous traumatic stress. A major message in this book is that unresolved trauma can result in unwanted symptoms. Ego State Therapy is precisely suited for work with clients suffering from PTSD symptoms. When the ego state that was traumatized is allowed expression, is encouraged to internally remove the threatening agent, and then receives internal help for whatever needs that persist, the unwanted symptoms of PTSD disappear. They are no longer driven by the angst of an underlying state that had carried unresolved trauma, a state that with ego state techniques has overcome fear, become empowered, and feels at ease. The application of Ego State Therapy techniques allows the therapist and client to focus directly on the residual trauma and resolve it by bringing out, and attending to, the specific state that holds that trauma. The reader should refer to the "Working with Trauma, 3.1" sections of this book for techniques that facilitate the cessation of PTSD symptoms.

Chapter 5

The Ego State Session

Should Ego State Therapy be used with every client? How is the therapy introduced to the client? What are the components of a typical ego state session? These are important questions that therapists need to consider in preparing to use Ego State Therapy. While the answers will vary, depending on the therapist and the client, the following section describes the processes that I adopt when using the therapy.

I use the therapy or theory with almost every client. Still, when a client comes in, I do not automatically think, "How can I apply Ego State Therapy here?" I listen to the client to discover what brought this person to therapy. As I hear the client describe the problem, I often hear it in relation to competing ego states, or in relation to some situational neurosis that may be connected to an earlier trauma. One of the advantages of Ego State Therapy is that I do not have to guess, or make an interpretation, about the cause of the problem. The cause will become evident when the affect bridge connects the problem with the cause.

Often clients will believe they know the cause and I will listen to their ideas, but I do not focus on their analysis of the situation since it has been my experience that they are often wrong. I do not share this view with my clients. I do not ask them "why" if they do not give a reason for their unwanted symptoms. "Why"s place the client in an intellectual state and problems that bring clients to therapy are almost always feeling based. Even when a person comes to counselling because of a difficulty in making a decision, it is the feeling of frustration that is troublesome. If a person cannot decide which color is he or she likes most, and if there is no anxiety with the indecision it is not seen as a major problem. If the person is tortured with the indecision, then a problem exists. It is important to hear what the problem is, not why the client thinks it exists.

I want to respond to the questions, "How is Ego State Therapy introduced to the client?" and "What are the components of a typical ego state session?" by presenting three typical ego state sessions. Each session corresponds with one of the main functions of the therapy.

5.1 Components of an Ego State Therapy Session

There are three general goals that may be achieved using Ego State Therapy. As stated at the beginning of the book, they are

1. to locate ego states harboring pain, trauma, anger, or frustration and facilitate release, empowerment and, comfort,
2. to facilitate functional communication between ego states, and
3. to allow clients to learn their ego states so they may be better used to the benefit of the client.

This section will illustrate common steps for each of these goals. These illustrations will be of little value to a reader who has not carefully read the previous chapters, as they are presented as an ordered summary of the more detailed techniques and theory. It should be noted that I do not advocate following a list of steps when working with clients. Each client is different. The best therapy is provided when the therapist learns techniques and hones skills, then enters the client's world and follows the path that fits that client at that time. The point of focus for the therapist should be with the client, not thinking about steps, or how the process is going. The combination of paying attention to the client, having a desire to help achieve a resolution, and having a tenacity to continue through dead ends generates the creativity needed for the best results. The following three subsections, therefore, are presented as an illustration of Ego State Therapy for each of the three general goals, not as a cookbook proscription to be followed, as the focus should always be with the client, not on the process being adopted. Some points are repeated in each section so the reader will not have to page back and forth while reading a session.

5.1.1 A Session to Resolve Trauma

Trauma resolution in Ego State Therapy corresponds to the goal of many psychodynamic therapies. A situational neurosis (the client is responding inappropriately to some situation in life) exists as a prerequisite for this technique, and the therapeutic intervention facilitates the discovery of the original trauma that fuels the neurosis, and facilitates the resolution of that original trauma, thus eliminating the neurosis. The following are normal components of this intervention:

1. Interview the client to discover the exact symptoms of the neurosis.
2. Introduce ego state theory.
3. Introduce hypnosis.
4. Ask if there are any questions about ego state theory, therapy, and hypnosis.
5. Use a hypnotic induction.
6. Near the end of the induction have the client focus on the symptomatic feelings of the neurosis.
7. Enhance the negative feelings until significant affect is demonstrated.
8. Re-stating the feelings, ask the client the age that is being experienced.
9. Ask the client, while experiencing those feelings, to return to that age when those feelings were first experienced.
10. Ask the client if he or she is inside or outside.
11. Ask the client if he or she is alone or with someone else.
12. Ask the client to describe exactly what is happening.
13. Facilitate the client to rise above fear and express true feelings to the antagonist.
14. Ask the client what else is needed in order to feel complete resolution.
15. Gain help for the traumatized state from other states that can help.
16. Check to make sure that all needs of the state have been met.
17. Express gratitude, by name, to all states that have spoken.
18. Ask the client to imagine being where the neurosis would have normally been experienced.
19. Check affect, to make sure the unwanted symptoms are not present.

20. If the unwanted symptoms are present go to 7 above and proceed.
21. Make sure no state is left with needs that cannot wait until the next session.
22. If the unwanted symptoms are not present, bring the client out of hypnosis.
23. Facilitate expression concerning the client's experience of the session.
24. End the session.

Each of the steps for trauma resolution will now be explained.

1. *Interview the client to discover the exact symptoms of the neurosis.* What is it that brought the client into therapy? Find out the goal of the client. What does the client want changed? If the client is presenting with a situational neurosis, trauma resolution is indicated. Clients who are having difficulty handling their emotions, clients who have difficulty handling particular aspects of their life, clients who do not understand why they respond in the way they do, will likely benefit from trauma resolution Ego State Therapy.

   Gather detailed information concerning a time when the client experienced the negative symptom. Take notes on the setting. Who else was present? What was the emotional and physical experience of the client? Find out what types of situation bring out these unwanted symptoms. The unwanted symptoms are the unprocessed aspects of an ego state that is coming to the executive during these times.

   It is very important that relevant and detailed information is gathered. You will be able to use the information you gather to bring the state needing resolution to the executive, to locate the origin of the trauma, and after process resolution, to check that the trauma has been resolved.

   It is not important to gather information concerning why the client believes the symptoms exist. If the client has a need to express reasoning it can build rapport to listen, but these reasons are often inaccurate, and the origin of the problem will be discovered within the process of Ego State Therapy.

2. *Introduce ego state theory.*
    It is not necessary to spend much time introducing ego state theory. If it is the first time the client has heard of Ego State Therapy it is helpful to describe the therapy. Useful information to relate in your own words in relation to the understanding of the client may include the following:

    We all have different states. They are very normal and enhance our experience of living by our being able to draw on states that have different strengths. Ego State Therapy allows therapy to progress quickly since the individual state that can benefit most is brought out and empowered. This process works best with the additional focus that hypnosis facilitates.

3. *Introduce hypnosis.*
    It is not necessary to spend much time talking about hypnosis. If the client has not been clinically hypnotized before it is good to share some information so unreal expectations do not interfere. Useful information to relate in your own words may include the following:

    Hypnosis is a normal state that we have each spontaneously experienced. Often, during hypnosis, people are completely aware of what is being said, and they may experience it as an increased ability to focus. It really does not matter the specific manner that you experience the feeling. You will be able to talk with me and express your thoughts and feelings.

4. *Ask if there are any questions about ego state theory, therapy, and hypnosis.*
    Make sure the client feels able to ask any questions about either Ego State Therapy or hypnosis. Respond fully to any questions, and ask if there are any further questions until all have been calmly addressed.

5. *Use a hypnotic induction.*
    Use any hypnotic induction you prefer. It is not necessary that a deep state be achieved before beginning therapy. The next step will deepen the level of hypnosis. Hypnosis will allow the client to have better access to underlying ego states. Without hypnosis, clients will have access only to surface ego states

(see section 2). Trauma resolution Ego State Therapy requires access to underlying ego states.

6. *Near the end of the induction have the client focus on the sympto-matic feelings of the neurosis.*
   This is where you first use the information gathered in step 1 above. Using the imagery the client has provided, place the client in the setting, with the emotional and physical sensa-tions the client has related. Use the client's own words to bring out the feelings of the unwanted symptom. Here, you are bringing out the ego state that needs resolution.

7. *Enhance the negative feelings until significant affect is demonstrated.*
   It is important for the client to show significant affect for the affect bridge or somatic bridge (using physical sensations rather than emotional feelings) to be effective. If the client is already demonstrating significant affect you can go strait to the next step. If the client is not demonstrating significant affect, deepen the affect.

   This increase in affect can normally be accomplished by ask-ing the client to report on a scale of 1 to 100 the intensity of the negative feeling (describe the feeling in detail to the client, just as it was described to you). Then ask the client if this feeling (name it again) can be increased to a higher number. Continue to have the client increase the intensity of the feeling until noticeable affect is demonstrated. In this process, do not say, "the feeling". Always describe the symptoms of the feeling, and do this with affect in your own voice. For example, rather than saying, "I wonder if you can increase that feeling?" it is better to say, "I wonder if you can increase that sense of being out of control?"

8. *Restating the feelings, ask the client the age that is being experienced.*
   Say something such as, "Feeling like you do right now, with (restate negative feelings), about how old do you feel, as you feel this way?"

9. *Ask the client, while experiencing those feelings, to return to that age when those feelings were first experienced.*
   Say something like, "Go right now to when you were about (answer of last question), having the feelings you are having right now of (restate negative feelings)." This takes the client to the original trauma

that has never been processed, that holds unresolved feelings that continue to surface for resolution. The following two questions help the client become more fully present in that trauma so processing can proceed. They should be asked in a rather rapid succession.

10. *Ask the client if he or she is inside or outside.*
    The client will normally have an awareness of being inside or outside. This helps the client zero in on the disturbance with giving any suggestions. Then go to the next question.

11. *Ask the client if he or she is alone or with someone else.*
    This question further facilitates the client to focus in on the original disturbance. After asking this question it is common that the client may be quite emotional. It is imperative that the client be allowed to be in this emotion so it may be resolved. It is the hypnotherapist's role to allow this emotion to be expressed, regardless of the level of affect. If you feel you are not able to be with a client who is experiencing severe affect, do not begin this line of questioning. It is better not to revisit a trauma, if the trauma is not going to be processed to a positive conclusion.

12. *Ask the client to describe exactly what is happening.*
    The client is now able to describe, in detail, what happened that started the situational neurosis. It is imperative that the client continues to stay in the ego state at the time that it was traumatized. This is a good time to ask this state what you can call it. You will want to be able to recall it at a later time.

13. *Facilitate the client to rise above fear and express true feelings to the antagonist.*
    The state has held onto fear since the original occurrence. It is this fear that reasserts itself when the negative experience is manifested. By expressing true feelings to the aggressor the fear is overcome.

    Sometimes a state is too frightened to be able to speak to the introject. When this is the case I offer to speak to the introject first. What I say depends on how the client has described the situation to me. Before speaking directly to the introject, the therapist should ask the client if this is alright, "Do you want me to tell him first?"

When speaking directly to the introject, speak loudly and with affect. Show the client that you are not afraid. Speak puni-tively, "You had no right to do what you did!!", then say to the client, "OK, now you can tell him. Tell him what you feel."

It is important that the client is able to personally say what is felt. This is integral in releasing fear.

14. *Ask the client what else is needed in order to feel complete resolution.* You can ask, "What do you need now?" or "What would make you feel better?" This will enable you to leave the state in an empowered and relaxed condition, as a state that will no longer carry distressed feelings that distress the client in par-ticular situations.

15. *Gain help for the traumatized state from other states that can help.* If a state says it needs a hug, you can ask to speak with a state that would like to help this state by giving it a hug. If it is lonely, you can ask to speak to a state that would like to stay with the needy state to keep it from being lonely. It is impor-tant to find states that 'want' to take on the helping role, rather than states that just agree to do it. When a state takes on a role it likes, it will continue with that role.

16. *Check to make sure that all needs of the state have been met.* This is accomplished by making sure that the state has expressed itself with everything it wants to say, and by mak-ing sure that it is not holding any negative or needy feelings. Resolution for that state is complete when the state is com-fortable and expresses satisfaction with how it feels.

17. *Express gratitude, by name, to all states that have spoken.* I like to say 'thank you' to each state I have spoken with, and show verbal appreciation by thanking each state for the tasks it has finished, or agreed to do. This also serves to clarify to the states the exact roles they will be having within the family of states.

18. *Ask the client to imagine being where the neurosis would have normally been experienced.*
    Use the client's example from question 1 above, of where and when the unwanted feelings would normally be experienced. Do not suggest feelings that the client might have. Rather, verbally place the client in the situation that would have previously brought out negative feelings.

19. *Check affect, to make sure the unwanted symptoms are not present.*
    After building the scene of the place that previously would have resulted in unwanted feelings, ask the client to report current feelings.

20. *If the unwanted symptoms are present go to 7 above and proceed.*
    Occasionally the ego state that gains resolution is not the ego state that becomes executive during the checking procedure. If this is the case, good work has still been accomplished, but more work is necessary. If there is time, you can go back to step 7 above, or if the session is near completion you may have to process these still unresolved feelings during the next session.

21. *Make sure no state is left with needs that cannot wait until the next session.*
    A good question to ask before ending an ego state session is, "Is there any part that has a something that needs attention right now?" Sometimes after working with states a part will be exposed in a way that demands immediate attention. If that part does not get its needs met at that time the client may feel a significant amount of distress in the short-term. It is therefore good to make sure that all parts are reasonably ready for the session to end. It must be the therapist's professional judgment that determines when to stop a session if several parts are needy.

22. *If the unwanted symptoms are not present, bring the client out of hypnosis.*
    Normally, the client will report no negative feelings when placed again in the situation that would have previously caused neurotic symptoms. If this is the case, this part of therapy is finished. It is good to debrief with the client again after

there has been a chance to check the effectiveness of the procedure outside of therapy.

23. *Facilitate expression concerning the client's experience of the session.* Debrief with clients. Ask them what they thought of their sessions. Ask if they have any questions. Take time to explain the theory, and how it works. Clients appreciate being informed.

24. *End the session.*

5.1.2   A Session to Enhance Internal Communication

It is only possible to feel generally settled and relaxed when there is good internal communication between ego states. There is likely poor internal communication or cooperation when the client does not like part of self, when the client feels split over major decisions, or when the client shows inconsistency in function.

A client saying, "I get so made at myself", is an example of a one ego state that does not like another ego state. "Sometimes I know I want to stay in school, and sometimes I know I don't want to stay in school", is an example of a client who feels split. Two ego states have not been able to agree. "Before I went into take the test I knew every answer, but when I sat down it was all gone", is an example of inconsistency in function. The most appropriate ego state is not taking the test.

Ego State Therapy can assist with these types of problems by facilitating an improvement in internal communication of states. First the steps for a session to improve internal communication will be listed then each will be briefly discussed:

1.   Interview the client to discover how the client is experiencing inner conflict.
2.   Introduce ego state theory.
3.   Introduce hypnosis.
4.   Ask if there are any questions about ego state theory, therapy, and hypnosis.
5.   Use a hypnotic induction.

6. Talk with one of the states that are involved with the internal conflict.
7. Talk with each of the other states involved with the conflict.
8. Determine if other states should also be involved by investigating internal resources.
9. Negotiate with all states, facilitating function changes (in degree) and trading.
10. Make sure all states 'prefer' the new arrangement.
11. Express gratitude, by name, to all states that have spoken.
12. Bring the client out of hypnosis.
13. Facilitate expression concerning the client's experience of the session.
14. End the session.

Each of the steps for improved internal communication will now be explained.

1. *Interview the client to discover how the client is experiencing inner conflict.*

   Find out what brought the client to therapy. If the cause is related to the inner conflict of ego states find out specifically how the symptoms are being experienced. Hear from both sides of the conflict. By doing this you are hearing from at least two ego states. Take specific notes on what each state has to say, in its own language. You will be able to use this information during the hypnosis session.

(Points 2–4 here are the same as in the trauma section.)

2. *Introduce ego state theory.*

   It is not necessary to spend much time introducing ego state theory. If it is the first time the client has heard of Ego State Therapy it is helpful to describe the therapy. Useful information to relate in your own words in relation to the understanding of the client may include the following:

   We all have different states. They are very normal and enhance our experience of living by our being able to draw on states that have different strengths. Ego State Therapy allows therapy to progress quickly since the individual state that can benefit most is brought out and empowered. This process works best with the additional focus that hypnosis facilitates.

3. *Introduce hypnosis.*
   It is not necessary to spend much time talking about hypnosis either. If the client has not been clinically hypnotized before it is good to share some information so unreal expectations do not interfere. Useful information to relate in your own words in relation to the understanding of the client may include the following.

   Hypnosis is a normal state that we have all spontaneously experienced. Often, during hypnosis, people are completely aware of what is being said, and they may experience it as an increased ability to focus. It really does not matter the specific manner that you experience the feeling. You will be able to talk with me and express your thoughts and feelings.

4. *Ask if there are any questions about ego state theory, therapy, and hypnosis.*
   Make sure the client feels able to ask any questions about either Ego State Therapy or hypnosis. Respond fully to any questions, and ask if there are any further questions until all have been calmly addressed.

5. *Use a hypnotic induction.*
   Use any hypnotic induction you prefer. It is not necessary that a deep state be achieved before beginning therapy. The next step will deepen the level of hypnosis. Hypnosis will allow the client to have better access to underlying ego states. Without hypnosis clients will have access only to surface ego states (see section 2). Working with surface states can resolve many areas of conflict within the client, but much conflict involves under-lying states. Using hypnosis greatly increases the power and effectiveness of Ego State Therapy.

6. *Talk with one of the states that are involved with the internal conflict.*
   Here you use some of the information you collected in step 1 above. Say to the hypnotized client that you want to speak with that part that believes or feels … (then use the language of the state that expressed itself in the first step). For example

you might say, "I want to talk with the part of you that gets really tired of all the study you have to do in school, the part that just wants to have your own time again."

If the inner conflict relates to states that don't like each other you can say something like, "I want to take with the state that is embarrassed by that part of you that sometimes expresses anger loudly."

This drawing out a state into conversation (bringing the state to the executive) is necessary for conflict resolution. Remember to talk with each state respectfully, and to talk about each state respectfully in order to maintain a good working relationship with all states (see section 2.2.2). Exhibit interest to hear what the state has to say. If another state jumps in with a "but on the other side" politely say that right now you want to continue to hear only from the one state. You can tell the other state that you will want to talk with it later.

7. *Talk with each of the other states involved with the conflict.*
   Next ask for the other state that you have gathered informa-tion from, for example, the angry state. Make sure you hold the state you want to speak with in the executive. If this seems very difficult, in other words if a different state really wants to talk, go ahead and hear what it has to say, than ask it politely if you can talk with 'the angry state' again.

   After you have heard what the two states have to say, ask if any other states have an opinion on the topic. "Is there any other part that would like to say something about the…?" Make sure you hear from all interested states, because these other states can sabotage an agreement if they are unhappy with it.

8. *Determine if other states should also be involved by investigating internal resources.*
   Sometimes you will need the help of states that have not shown an interest in the outcome. For example, if you are negotiating between a state that is upset and embarrassed by an overtly, loud, angry state, and the state that shows loud anger, it may be helpful to enlist the help of a state that can be assertive. An assertive state may be enlisted to release pent-up

anxiety so the state that expresses anger does not have to. A three-way negotiation may resolve the problem to the satisfaction of all states.

9. *Negotiate with all states, facilitating function changes (in degree) and trading.*
   The assertive state may be asked if it would be willing to take on a larger role, and continue to release anxiety assertively. The state that can become angry may be ask if it would be willing to allow the assertive state to take on this larger role, so it could step in and express real anger only when it is really appropriate. The state that was upset with the anger state may be ask if it is willing to respect and appreciate the state that can express anger, if it takes this more confined role. A wise state may be called upon to determine when anxiety is best released by the assertive state, and when it is best released by the state that can express anger.

   All states should be encouraged to confirm agreements with each other internally, and the process is not finished until all states are happy with the outcome. Creativity is often beneficial in negotiating these internal conflicts.

10. *Make sure all states 'prefer' the new arrangement.*
    If one of the states is not happy with the agreement changes will probably not be lasting. When all states are happy with the agreement it rarely does not last. One factor that helps facilitate internal agreements is that states enjoy being liked by other states. It is common in the initial stages of a negotiation among states for a state to say, "I don't care what they think of me", when referring to other states that have not liked that state. When agreements are made and states can see they are accepted and appreciated by other states they soften and often express feeling positive about being accepted. A good negotiating technique is to say to a state that has not been liked in the past, "Wouldn't it be good if the other states could appreciate how important you are, and how much need there is for what you can do?"

    The process of negotiation is finished when all states are happy with the outcome. The therapist should show respect for all states throughout the negotiation, and encourage states to appreciate the functions of each. An important question to ask before ending the session is, "Are there any states that have anything that needs to be said?" This question allows a state that may have unmet needs to express those needs.

11. *Express gratitude, by name, to all states that have spoken.*
    I like to say 'thank you' to each state I have spoken with, and show verbal appreciation by thanking each state for the tasks it has finished, or agreed to do. This also serves to clarify to the states the exact roles they will be having within the family of states.

12. *Bring the client out of hypnosis.*
    Before ending the hypnosis session I like to ask one more time if any other state has anything it needs to say. Sometimes this question is not possible if another client is waiting, because it can result in a longer session, but when possible it acts as an additional check that the process is finished and the positive outcome will last.

13. *Facilitate expression concerning the client's experience of the session.*
    Debrief with clients. Ask them what they thought of their sessions. Ask if they have any questions. Take time to explain the theory, and how it works. Clients appreciate being informed.

14. *End the session.*

5.1.3 A Session to Promote Self Awareness and Knowledge of Strengths

Understanding who we are and why we are the way we are is enhanced with ego state mapping. Clients can learn their parts and benefit from being able to call to the executive ego states with strengths that match the requirements of the moment. Ego state mapping is an integral part of couples counselling (see section 4.3). The following is an example of a session to increase this self-awareness and knowledge of strengths.

1. Interview the client to discover the detail of ego state mapping preferred.

2.   Ask the client to specify any particular areas where improved function is desired.
3.   Introduce ego state theory.
4.   Introduce hypnosis.
5.   Ask if there are any questions about ego state theory, therapy, and hypnosis.
6.   Gather information about two different mood states.
7.   Use a hypnotic induction.
8.   Use the information gathered about the mood states to bring one state to the executive.
9.   Talk with the first state, then bring to the executive the other state, using the information gathered prior to hypnosis.
10. Switch back and forth between the two states.
11. Talk with other states, gathering information from each.
12. Call for other states that the client has expressed a functional desire to use.
13. Keep excellent notes.
14. Express gratitude, by name, to all states that have spoken.
15. Bring the client out of hypnosis.
16. Discuss the states with the client and discuss with the client ways they may be used to advantage.
17. Facilitate expression concerning the client's experience of the session.
18. End the session.
19. Create a clear ego state map for the client and for your records.

Each of the steps to promote self-awareness and knowledge of strengths will now be explained.

1.   *Interview the client to discover the detail of ego state mapping preferred.*
     Part of this session will entail educating the client concerning the options (see section 3.3.5). Depending on the detail preferred by the client the number of mapping sessions will range from one to several.

2.   *Ask the client to specify any particular areas where improved function is desired.*
     It is the role of the therapist to bring resources to needs. Therefore, it is important to understand precisely what areas the client wants to focus upon. For example, if the client wants

to focus on ego states that have more to do with performance at work, states that might impact upon that performance could be mapped. If the client wants to focus on personal relationships ego states that may impact in that area could be the primary focus.

(Points 3, 4, 5, and 7 here are the same as points 2–5 in the trauma section.)

3. *Introduce ego state theory.*
   It is not necessary to spend much time introducing ego state theory. If it is the first time the client has heard of Ego State Therapy it is helpful to describe the therapy. Useful information to relate in your own words in relation to the understanding of the client may include the following:

   We all have different states. They are very normal and enhance our experience of living by our being able to draw on states that have different strengths. Ego State Therapy allows therapy to progress quickly since the individual state that can benefit most is brought out and empowered. This process works best with the additional focus that hypnosis facilitates.

4. *Introduce hypnosis.*
   It is not necessary to spend much time talking about hypnosis either. If the client has not been clinically hypnotized before it is good to share some information so unreal expectations do not interfere. Useful information to relate in your own words in relation to the understanding of the client may include the following:

   Hypnosis is a normal state that we have all spontaneously experienced. Often, during hypnosis, people are completely aware of what is being said, and they may experience it as an increased ability to focus. It really does not matter the specific manner that you experience the feeling. You will be able to talk with me and express your thoughts and feelings.

5. *Ask if there are any questions about ego state theory, therapy, and hypnosis.*
   Make sure the client feels able to ask any questions about either Ego State Therapy or hypnosis. Respond fully to any questions, and ask if there are any further questions until all have been calmly addressed.

6. *Gather information about two different mood states.*
   Discuss with the client at least two different states, for example for a particular person, gather information about a state that feels out of control with children, and about a state that feels in control with a close friend. These states should be specific to the client. Information should be gathered relating to these states, such as where the client experienced them, with whom, the feelings experienced, the sensory perceptions; information that will enable you to "assist the client into the experience of the state while under hypnosis".

7. *Use a hypnotic induction.*
   Use any hypnotic induction you prefer. It is not necessary that a deep state be achieved before beginning therapy. The next step will deepen the level of hypnosis. Hypnosis will allow the client to have better access to underlying ego states. Without hypnosis clients will have access only to surface ego states (see section 2). Working with surface states can resolve many areas of conflict within the client, but much conflict involves underlying states. Using hypnosis greatly increases the power and effectiveness of Ego State Therapy.

8. *Use the information gathered about the mood states to bring one state to the executive.*
   Here you bring to the executive one of the states the client described prior to hypnosis. Do this by mentioning scenes the client has spoken about using the client's own words, like "You're setting on the brown couch with your feet curled up under you, the light is dim with the red candle bringing light in from the left. Your friend Joan is smiling and sitting in the beige chair across from you. You're feeling very relaxed and able to speak easily."

9. *Talk with the first state, then bring to the executive the other state, using the information gathered prior to hypnosis.*
    As you place the client into the scene where the ego state you want to speak with is normally executive, begin to speak directly to this state: "With your friend sitting across from you there, with the light coming from the red candle on the coffee table, how are you feeling?" Ask this state what you can call it: "Feeling relaxed as you are, there talking with you friend, what can I call this part of you?" Say "thank you" to the first state (in this example it named itself 'Relaxed', see section 2.2.2) for talking with you and tell it you will want to speak to it again. "Thank you 'Relaxed", I will want to talk with you again, but right now I want to speak with that part of you that is talking with your children, and they are not listening." Bring the second state to the executive, as described in step 8 above. Talk with the second state and get a name for it, as you did for the first state.

10. *Switch back and forth between the two states.*
    Continue to speak with these two states, calling them by name and switching back and forth between them. When you want to talk with a state you have already spoken with, call it by name. "'Relaxed", I want to speak with you now. Just say 'I'm here' when you are ready to speak." As the conversation progresses you will be able to bring states back to the executive easily, "Relaxed, did you hear that?" or "Relaxed, what do you think of that?"

11. *Talk with other states, gathering information from each.*
    Once the client is easily switching between the first two states other states are normally easy to access. There are several ways to access other states. You can ask a state you are speaking with, "What other states do you know?" (See section 2.2.2), then call those states out. You can ask to speak with a state that has a specific function, "I would like to talk with a part of you that is nurturing, a state that likes to help others, children or adults." You may notice the client automatically switching. When this happens show acknowledgement, "This isn't relaxed I'm talking with now, is it? What part am I talking with now?" You can ask to talk with a state that has some knowledge about a certain topic, "I would like to talk with the state that is really good at sitting quietly and writing."

191

12. *Call for other states that the client has expressed a functional desire to use.*

    If the client has previously expressed a desire to be more assertive, it is important to ask to speak with a state that can be assertive. It is sometimes the case that no state is quick to come forward, when asked. You may have to continue to encourage a needed state to come to the executive, "There may be a part of you that has been assertive in the past, possibly with a child, or with a really pushy person. I would like to talk with that state that has been able to be expressive. Just say, 'I'm here' when you are ready to talk."

    When a state has been called to the executive and has spoken in the executive, the client will become familiar with that state, and will be able to bring it out later with it is needed.

13. *Keep excellent notes.*

    Make sure you get a name for each state. It is a good idea to circle state names so they can be quickly and easily seen on the page. Write down the traits and functions of each state. Write down how the states work together. For a particular client, a 'fear' state may work with an 'anger' state, and call it to the executive when the need exists. These notes will be needed to create an ego state map for the client later.

14. *Express gratitude, by name, to all states that have spoken.*

    After speaking with several states, including those states that pertain specifically with the needs expressed by the client, refer to your notes and thank, by name, each state you have spoken with. "I want to thank 'Relaxed' and 'Troubled' and … All the states can now go where they need to go." By showing respect to all states they will be anxious to talk with you again if the need arises, and they may be more cooperative when called upon by the client. Ego State Therapy should be a good experience for the client, the therapist, and for each state within the client. While some techniques of Ego State Therapy involve processing painful trauma, if techniques are applied with skill and sensitivity each state should be able to experience the outcome as positive.

15. *Bring the client out of hypnosis.*
    Before ending the hypnosis session I like to ask if any state has anything it needs to say. Sometimes this question is not possible if another client is waiting, because it can result in a longer session, but when possible it acts as an additional check that the process is finished and will the outcome is positive.

16. *Discuss the states with the client and discuss with the client ways they may be used to advantage.*
    Using the notes you have taken, debrief with the client concerning the nature of the states, and how the states may be called to the executive for use in the future. Discuss each state in a positive way. Remind the client about how the states work together, using the client's specific states in the discussion.

17. *Facilitate expression concerning the client's experience of the session.*
    Debrief with clients. Ask them what they thought of their sessions. Ask if they have any questions. Take time to explain the theory, and how it works. Clients appreciate being informed.

18. *End the session.*

19. *Create a clear ego state map for the client and for your records.*
    When the purpose of Ego State Therapy is to facilitate growth by mapping the ego states it is useful to create a clear ego state map for the client. Circle the names of the ego states. This map will usually be able to be placed on a single page. Ego states that work together may be placed close together on the page. Ego states that communicate with each other may be connected by a line. Aspects of each state may be written under the name. Depending on the needs of the client it may be helpful to have a session to present the ego state map, discuss it, and discuss how it may be used to the benefit of the client.

    During an ego state mapping session states that hold trauma or states that have state-to-state communication difficulties may become evident. When this occurs I make sure that the client is interested in dealing with these issues in counselling before proceeding toward a resolution. If the client has come only for mapping, deeper therapeutic work should not be started without direction from the client.

Chapter 6

Final Thoughts

Cognitive Behavioral Therapy is the most widely used therapy. This section addresses the question, "Why use Ego State Therapy rather than CBT?" Also discussed in this final section are some theoretical implications of ego state theory, in relation to the nature/nurture debate and in relation to the idea that individuals may experience false or blocked memories. The section, and the book, ends with some thoughts concerning the nature and value of Ego State Therapy.

6.1 Why Ego State Therapy?

Why do we need Ego State Therapy? Why not use CBT or some other therapy? Ego State Therapy is very fast and powerful and it provides a causal solution, not a coping strategy. It provides both direct access to the problem and it provides a means to change the state that has carried toxic trauma, pain, frustration, misunderstanding, or anger, to a state that can feel relieved, empowered and appreciated.

There is a place for Cognitive Behavioral Therapy in assisting clients. Often CBT techniques mixed with ego state techniques can speed the process of therapy. When a problem that brings a client to therapy is based in a trauma of the past, is based in an internal conflict between states, or could be alleviated by greater access to little used states, CBT is not enough.

CBT does not address issues from the past, does not facilitate causal solutions, and may provide merely a coping technique, leaving the injured self still injured. There is no doubt that it works to help the client better cope with situations they believe are beyond their control. Many studies reveal that clients using CBT are able to leave therapy with their goals largely addressed. Is that enough?

It is feelings that define us as human. Feelings touch our souls and bring richness to life. When a part of our psyche is injured, traumatized, and frail, we avoid it and hide from it. We learn to live a task-oriented, detached existence. To paste a coping skill on the surface of an injured personality is to further remove that person emotionally from self. The further we are removed from our beautiful child states, which are able to feel deeply, which are able to feel love and wonder, the more like a robot or computer we become. We learn to function and go on, but do we learn to live more richly? Improving mental health is being able to re-enter that fragile center part and feel deeply.

CBT became popular partly because it provided a quick solution compared to psychoanalysis and humanists therapies. Ego State Therapy provides a quick solution compared to CBT, and its solution is a causal solution, not a symptom solution. This means that while CBT therapists focus on the unwanted symptom and train the client to respond in a different way, ego state therapists use unwanted symptoms to locate the causal disturbance.

When the causal trauma is located and resolved, the symptom disappears. The symptom disappears along with the trauma. The trauma is no longer present to cause other problems, or to be experienced as an internal, unsettling disturbance. Internal ego states are cleared of fear, and this allows them to experience positive emotions. The client is able to feel integrated, more alive, and more able to enjoy living. An example may be illustrative.

A twenty-six-year-old client presented with the problem of not being able to enjoy anything connected with sexually amorous behavior. She reported that she had always hated sexual intercourse, and that even when her partner said sexually positive and sensitive things to her she became extremely upset. She had friends who talked positively about their sexual experiences and she felt she was missing out on what could be a very positive part of her life with her partner.

An affect bridge was used to discover the origin of her problem. Some of the descriptions she used when talking about her feelings during foreplay were, "I just hate it. I feel like something is pressing down on me, like I just want to break away. I don't know if

I am angry, but I don't like it." The emotions were heightened and the affect bridge (see section 2.2.5) took her to a time when she was 10 years old. Two older cousins were raping her. (This was a memory she had always had, but she had not thought it related to her problem.) She cried loudly, and while she was in that injured state I asked her to tell her cousins what she wanted to tell them. She was, for the first time, able to express herself to the perpetrators. The 10-year-old state was able to yell at them and release feelings that had been held for 16 years. With ego state work the 10-year-old state was able to feel supported and understood. It gained resolution, no longer feeling fearful with an absence of completion.

After the hypnosis I used a behavioral technique as an adjunct to the ego state work. I asked her to arrange with her partner that for, as long as she felt appropriate, she would be the director of any sexual encounters. She would decide the speed and the degree of any sexual encounters, and she was further asked to think of herself as a teenager discovering sex for the first time. Her partner was glad to agree.

Four weeks later she reported much pleasure in their sexual activities. She said it was fantastic, and she could not believe what she had missed for so long. She was surprised that the rape she had mentally dismissed could have had such a long and profound impact on her. That unresolved, injured part had previously returned whenever it was reminded of the original occurrence. It returned with its feelings and experiences of that occurrence.

The focus of the treatment was on the cause, the rape. We knew the rape was the cause, not because of what she had thought, but because the affect bridge led us there. When the 10-year-old state was able to gain the resolution it needed, then the adult was able to respond in a sexual relationship without interference.

A CBT intervention would have focused on the symptom. She may have been asked to think about sex differently, to systematically take sex very slowly until she could function without so much anxiety, or to accept that not everyone enjoys sex and there is nothing wrong with that. She might have been able to perform sexually with less anxiety than she had experienced previously, but she would not have been able to feel free of the internal trauma that was inappropriately associated with sexually amorous behavior. She would have continued to carry the unresolved 10-year-old state, and this state would have continued to be part of her experience of life, manifesting itself in some way. Fear associated with that state would have prevented her from many joyous experiences.

Ego State Therapy focuses on the cause, and by resolving the cause the symptoms disappear. It is a brief therapy with lasting results.

6.2   Theoretical Implications of Ego State Theory

Ego state theory is more than a theory of therapy. It is also a theory of personality. The assumption that the personality is composed of a grouping of separate states, each possessing identity, memory, and specific traits, defines the personality structure. Ego states are created according to need, and continue to be active, or available to varying degrees. Unresolved trauma produces a tension that may continue to interrupt normal function. Internal state-to-state communication problems may interfere with individual's ability to relax and feel at peace.

Ego state personality theory has implications relating to some of our basic understandings of the nature of the mind. This section briefly examines the implications of ego state theory on our understandings of false memories and the nature-nurture debate.

6.2.1   Blocked and False Memories

Recently a debate in the literature centers has begun on memories of early trauma, memories that the client does not report recalling prior to adulthood. The debate centers on the validity of these late onset memories. Some authors believe that a traumatic experience will be remembered throughout life and a late onset memory of a traumatic event will likely be a false memory. Other authors believe that almost all late onset memories represent real occurrences; they believe that these memories were previously blocked.

Hypnotherapy used with coercive suggestion can result in the creation a false memory, so it is difficult to pose an argument that false memories do not exist. Even without hypnosis, confused memories about aspects of our past are more the rule than the exception. It appears that hypnotically recovered memories (without coercive suggestion) have about the same validity as normal memories; that is, mainly accurate, but with mistakes.

We can be equally certain that, although false memories are a feature of our recall, late onset memories can be accurate. Real memories can be blocked, or at least temporarily forgotten. Hypnosis is often able to assist a client to recall events that occurred and that are, at least sometimes, verifiable. A person suffering from Dissociative Identity Disorder (Multiple Personality) may not remember what he or she was doing five minutes before, when in a different alter. This is an example of a state having no memory of an earlier occurrence, and it substantiates the argument that late onset memories can be valid.

There is a real difficulty when a client has a late onset memory of childhood abuse and the abuser vehemently denies ever being an abuser. The problem is, it may be impossible to discover if the memory is a real memory that has been blocked, or if the memory is a false memory that has been generated by suggestion, life circumstance, or expectation. Is the accused guilty of abuse, or a loving parent improperly accused? This is a difficult question and may never be able to be completely resolved. There is no way to distinguish a false memory from a real one. Hypnosis cannot distinguish these memories and Ego State Therapy cannot distinguish them.

Ego state theory allows a better understanding of the possibility that late onset memories are real, or false. Each person is dissociated to some degree along a continuum ranging from an extreme low level of dissociation to a very high level of dissociation. Those at the highest end of this continuum suffer dissociative identity disorder. It appears that a precursor to this disorder is chronic and severe child abuse, where over time the child unconsciously learns to forget the trauma after changing states, as a means of coping. This shutting down of communication between states causes the person to become near totally amnesic between certain, even surface, states. When a multiple is asked, "Were you ever abused in childhood?" the answer is often sincerely given, "No". The state answering the question may have no knowledge of any abuse because the state that suffered the abuse has no communication with this answering state. When the therapist speaks directly with the alter that experienced the abuse, graphic and horrific detail may be given. The more dissociated a person is, the more likely major life events will not be recalled.

The average person would fall near the center of the dissociation continuum. This person will be able to notice real changes in mood and states according to daily life circumstance, but will have good memories of any major events that occurred. Remember, we have surface states and underlying states. Our surface states are normally aware of our experiences, and only some underlying states may be unaware. While underlying states may hold detailed and specific memories of events that happened in our childhood, if an event was of major significance surface states will hold at least parts of that memory, unless higher levels of dissociation are part of the personality structure.

Those persons with less dissociation than average may find it difficulty to notice mood changes, or any ego state changes. They may be less able to experience the latitude of emotional and intellectual expression common with the general population. These individuals will have good memory covering the full range of childhood years. Their ego states exchange information freely and are almost indistinguishable. While they miss out on the more full range of states the average person enjoys, it is almost impossible for these persons not to recall any major event that occurred after early childhood.

Persons at any location along the dissociation continuum may have inaccurate and false memories. Ego state theory therefore allows us some insight into which late onset memories may more likely be true or false. Individuals toward the dissociative end of the continuum may have many late onset memories that are accurate, as states that experienced those events first hand find their way to the executive. An increase in communication between the states that experienced trauma and other states may result in many accurate late onset memories continuing to come into consciousness. Still, false memories are possible with this group, and as stated above there is no way to distinguish a false memory from a real one. The likelihood that late onset memories are true is at its highest with the more dissociative clients.

The less dissociative the client, the less likely late onset memories will be accurate. The higher level of communication between states with clients of average and below average levels of dissociation means that major events will most likely be recalled throughout the life span. It is unlikely that a late onset memory of a major event will be valid if the client has below average levels of dissociation. Indeed, since traumatic events lead to dissociation, and since dissociative identity disorder is associated with the chronic experience of traumatic events, a low level of dissociation, itself, is the likely result of a non-eventful childhood.

6.2.2 Nature/Nurture

What are the theoretical implications of ego states? If our individual psyche is the map of ego states we have developed during our life, what are the implications in terms of the nature-nurture debate? Scientists have long debated the amount of psyche that is attributed to nature (how we were born) verses nurture (the events in our life). Few cling to the notion that we are totally dictated by either, that who we will be is already decided at birth, or that we are a blank slate at birth; rather most believe we are the culmination of some level of the combination of the two. We are born with predispositions that can be modified along a range that was set at birth, and that modification is dependent upon our environment.

Proponents of the nature camp believe that range to be rather small. They would argue that our environment has a relatively small impact on whom we become. They point to identical twin studies that show the similarities of twins who were raised in different families, families that did not know of the existence of the other identical twin.

Proponents of the nurture camp believe that range to be rather large. They believe that environment is the major factor in determining who we will become. They point to evidence that shows the impact of parental nurturing.

Ego state theory appears to lend credence to the nurture side of the debate, at least in terms of much of our psychological experience of life. While nature may impact heavily on our intelligence, and possibly on our level of conservatism and energy, our situational neurosis are the result of our nurture, the things that happen in our life. This is not entirely the case.

Some children may be more 'nature' prone to experience trauma. On the first day of kindergarten there will be children who are excited about the new experience, and others who experience trauma. Practically any parent with more than a single child will talk about how their children were different from birth in the manner they experience life events. We appear predisposed to experience trauma in our own way. Of course, there are some experiences that would be traumatic to any child. Even these experiences are internalized in an individual fashion.

The important aspect of this discussion is that all children experience trauma. When trauma is experienced, it is best when it can be processed immediately after the experience. Like the name we know and cannot remember, and we cannot let go, unresolved trauma cannot be let go. It lies in waiting. An ego state with unresolved trauma will come forward when an occurrence presents itself that is similar to the original occurrence. It will come forward with the need for resolution. Ego State Therapy provides a theoretical framework to understand that need, and a process that enables therapists to help met that need for resolution.

6.3   Conclusion

Ego State Therapy has been presented in this book with techniques and examples relating to various applications. The personality is composed of several components, with each, when conscious, possessing its own ego identity. These ego state identities can be viewed as surface states (the states that commonly assume consciousness) and underlying states (states that seldom or never assume consciousness). Hypnosis allows verbal access to both surface and underlying ego states. Ego state access is useful in therapy in a number of ways. Underlying states may hold unresolved trauma that interferes in the life of the client, psychologically or physically. Internal arguments among states can result in distressful feelings when ego states cannot agree on what is best for the person. Ego states may have assumed roles for which they are not well suited. For example, an insecure state may assume consciousness for public speaking. Ego State Therapy is well suited for the resolution of all of these state dysfunctions, and it also allows an enhancement of ego state usage by providing the client with knowledge and access of various states. Clients may become aware of their particular ego state map so they can learn to access emotional, logical, or talent specific states (e.g., assertive, work focused, fun loving) to meet needs.

Ego State Therapy has grown and evolved since the mid-1970s and appears poised for development in several areas. The importance of training in hypnosis may inhibit some therapist from gaining he benefits of using this therapy, although it is anticipated that as the power and brevity of Ego State Therapy becomes better known, more therapists will undertake training in hypnosis. Ego State Therapy has been shown in this book to be especially useful for work with panic attack, psychosomatic symptoms, pain, drug addiction, dissociative identity disorder, depression, anger, and work with couples. It is most useful for finding and resolving unresolved trauma that has afflicted the client, often, since childhood (most usually without the client having an understanding of the origin of the problem).

It is hoped that this book will contribute to a better understanding of ego states, and enhance therapeutic practice. It is also hoped that it will inspire additional research and development in this powerful, brief therapy. Ego State Therapy has the potential to reclaim and enrich lives in a manner that nurtures understanding and appreciation of the family of states that lies within. To know our states is to know ourselves. The resolution of pain and trauma is healing. To achieve internal respect and collegiality fosters peace with self. What better achievement can we have as therapists than to help clients resolve the cause of their pain, to gain self-understanding, and to value themselves?

Bibliography

Beahrs, J. O., 1982, *Unity and multiplicity: Multilevel consciousness of self in hypnosis, psychiatric disorder and mental health*, Brunner/Mazel, New York.

Berne, E., 1961, *Transactional Analysis in Psychotherapy*, Grove Press.

Cady, R. K., & Farmer, K., 1993, *Headache Free*, Moray Press, Springfield, MO.

Caul, D., 1984, Group and videotape techniques for multiple personality disorder, *Psychiatric Annals*, **14**, 43–50.

Davidson, P., 1987, *Hypnosis and migraine headache: Reporting a clinical series*, **15**, 111–118.

Emmerson, G. J. & Farmer, K., 1996, Ego State Therapy and menstrual migraine, *The Australian Journal of Clinical Hypnotherapy & Hypnosis*, **17**, 7–14.

Emmerson G. J., 1987, *A Psychological Analysis of the Effects Indirect Induction Hypnosis, Imagery, and Suggestion Have on Goal Achievement*, UMI Dissertations, Ann Arbor, Michigan.

Emmerson, G. J., 1999, What lies within: ego states and other internal personifications, *The Australian Journal of Clinical Hypnotherapy and Hypnosis*, **20**, 13–22.

Emmerson, G. J., May 2000, Advanced Methods in Hypnotic Practice, *Australian Society of Clinical Hypnosis workshop* conducted at Northbrook House, East Malvern, Victoria, Australia.

Federn, P., 1952, *Ego psychology and the psychoses*, E. Weiss (ed.), Basic Books, New York.

Frederick, C., & McNeal, S., 1999, From strength to strength: "Inner strength" with immature ego states, *American Journal of Clinical Hypnosis*, **33**, 250–256.

Freud, S., 1901/1960, *Psychopathology of everyday life*. Hogarth Press, London.

Fricton J. R. & Roth, P., 1985, The Effects of Direct and Indirect Hypnotic Suggestions for Analgesia in High and Low Susceptible Subjects, *American Journal of Clinical Hypnosis*, 27, pp. 226-231.

Gainer, M. J., 1993, Somatization of dissociated traumatic memories in a case of reflex sympathetic dystrophy, *American Journal of Clinical Hypnosis*, **36**, 124–131.

Harding H. C., 1978, *Workshop on hypnotic treatment of migraine and obesity*, Queensland Branch of the Australian Society for Clinical and Experimental Hypnosis, Brisbane.

Hilgard, E., 1975, Hypnosis Section of Vol. 26 of the *Annual Review of Psychology*, pp. 19-44.

Hilgard, E. R., & Hilgard, J. R., 1975, *Hypnosis in the relief of Pain*. William Kaufmann, Los Altos, CA.

Jung, C. G., 1970, *Analytical psychology: Its theory and practice*, Random House, New York.

Moreno, J. L., 1946, *Psychodrama: First Volume*, Beacon House, Ambler, PA.

Newey, A. B., 1986, Ego State Therapy with depression, in B. Zilbergeld, M. G. Edelstien, & D. L. Araoz (eds.), *Hypnosis: Questions and answers*, Norton, New York, pp. 197–203.

Nores, J., Yakovleff, A., & Nenna, A. D., 1989, Some problems involving perception under anesthesia: The contribution of hypnosis to the understanding of the ego.

Perls, F. S., 1969, *Gestalt therapy verbatim*, Real People Press, Lafayette, CA.

Watkins, H. H., 1978, Ego State Therapy, in J. G. Watkins (ed.), *The Therapeutic Self*, Human Sciences, New York, pp. 360-398.

Watkins, H. H., 1980, The Silent Abreaction, *International Journal of Clinical and Experimental Hypnosis*, XXVIII, 101-113.

Watkins, J. G., 1949, *Hypnotherapy of War Neuroses*, Ronald, New York.

Watkins, J. G., 1971, The affect bridge: A hypnoanalytic technique, *International Journal of Clinical and Experimental Hypnosis*, **19**, 21–27.

Watkins, J. G., 1976, Ego States and the Problem of Responsibility: A Psychological Analysis of the Patty Hearst case, *Journal of Psychiatry and Law*, 471-489.

Watkins, J. G., 1977, The Psychodynamic Manipulation of Ego States in Hypnotherapy, in F. Antonelli (ed.), *Therapy in Psychsomatic Medicine*, Vol II, pp. 389-403, Symposia, Rome, Italy.

Watkins, J. G., 1978a, *The Therapeutic Self*, Human Sciences, New York.

Watkins, J. G., 1978b, Ego States and the Problem of Responsibility: A Psychological Analysis of Patricia W., *Journal of Psychiatry and Law*, 519-535.

Watkins, J. G., 1993, Dealing with the problem of false memory in clinic and court, *The Journal of Psychiatry & Law/Fall 1993*, 297 – 317

Watkins, J. G., 2000, Personal Communication, June, Missoula, Montana.

Watkins, J. G. & Watkins, H. H., 1976, *Hypnoanalytic ego-state therapy*, audio tape no. 97, American Academy of Psychotherapists Tape Library, Orlando, Florida.

Watkins, J. G., & Watkins, H. H., 1978, *The therapeutic self*, Human Sciences Press, New York.

Watkins, J. G., & Watkins, H. H., 1979a, Theory and Practice of Ego State Therapy: A Short-Term Therapeutic Approach, in H. Grayson (ed.), *Short term approaches to psychotherapy*, Human Sciences Press, New York, pp. 176-220.

Watkins, J. G. & Watkins, H. H., 1979b, Ego States and Hidden Observers. II. Ego State, *Journal of Altered States of Consciousness*, 5, 3-18.

Watkins, J. G. & Watkins, H. H., 1979c, Ego States and Hidden Observers. II. Ego State Therapy, *The Lady in White and the Woman in Black*, audio tape, Jeffrey Norton, New York.

Watkins, J. G., & Watkins, H. H., 1981, Ego State Therapy, in R. J. Corsini (ed.), *Handbook of innovative psychotherapies*, Wiley-Interscience, New York, pp. 252–270.

Watkins, J. G., & Watkins, H. H., 1982, Ego State Therapy, in L. E. Abt & I. R. Stuart (eds.), *The newer therapies: A sourcebook*, Van Nostrand Reinhold, New York, pp. 137–155.

Watkins, J. G., & Watkins, H. H., 1986, Hypnosis, multiple personality and ego states as altered states of consciousness, in B. W. Wolman & M. Ullman (eds.), *Handbook of states of consciousness*, Van Nostrand Reinhold, New York.

Watkins, J. G., & Watkins, H. H., 1988, The management of malevolent ego states in multiple personality disorder, Dissociation, **1**, 67–72.

Watkins, J. G., & Watkins, H. H., 1990, Dissociation and displacement: Where goes the "ouch?", *American Journal of Clinical Hypnosis*, **33**, 1–10.

Watkins, J. G., & Watkins, H. H., 1997, Ego states: *Theory and Therapy*, Norton, New York.

Weiss, E., 1960, *The Structure and Dynamics of the Human Mind*, Grunne & Statton, New York.

What is Psychosynthesis?, 2000, World Wide Web, http://www.chebucto.ns.ca/Health/Psychosynthesis/what/ps2.htm.

What is Voice Dialogue?, 2000, World Wide Web, http://voicedialogue.com/whatis.htm#top%20of%20page.

Glossary

Abreaction: A negative emotional or physical response in therapy that is related to an earlier trauma. Abreactions may occur while working through a trauma. In ego state theory, the act of experiencing an abreaction is not therapeutic, but the act of resolving the trauma, which often entails abreactions, is therapeutic. When a trauma is resolved no further abreactions associated with that trauma will occur. A panic attack can be thought of as an abreaction outside of therapy.

Affect Bridge: The affect bridge is a technique for discovering the origin to a neurotic symptom so a process of resolution can be initiated. Unwanted symptomatic emotions are brought to the experience of the hypnotized client followed by questioning concerning those feelings and a request for the client to return to the first time those feelings were experienced.

Alter: An alter is a personality state of a person with dissociative identity disorder (multiple personality). While surface ego states of a non-pathological individual communicate well with each other, allowing the person to have relatively continuous daily memory, 'alters' communicate poorly with each other, resulting in memory blackouts relating to times that other alters were executive.

Autonomic Finger Signal: In hypnosis autonomic finger signaling is a finger movement in response to a question, such as, "If you can hear me, move your right index finger." Occasionally a hypnotized person will be able to communicate with autonomic finger signaling when they cannot verbally.

Creative Form Identity (CFI): Creative form identities are much like ego states, with the difference being the physical form they report speaking from. They most usually speak with the identity of a body form, such as the left hand, the chest, the neck, or any body part or location. With Ego State Therapy the left hand may have a conversation with the right hand. It appears that creative form identities are actually ego states that use creative forms as a way of identifying themselves. Less normally than using a body part as an identifier, they report being a form such as a fish, or a bird.

Dissociative Identity Disorder (Multiple Personality): A psychological disorder assumed to be caused by chronic childhood abuse. Normal personality segments (ego states) lose their ability to communicate with each other, becoming alters. An alter will often have no memory of the times other alters were executive.

Ego State: An ego state is one of a group of similar states, each distinguished by particular role, mood and mental function, which when conscious assumes first person identity. Ego states are a normal part of a healthy psyche, and should not be confused with alters (multiple personalities in dissociative identity disorder).

Executive: An ego state or alter is said to be executive when it is conscious and able to communicate or function external to the individual. For example, a state speaking with another person, petting a dog, or washing a car is executive. Some non-executive states will be able to hear a conversation while others will not, but only one state is in the executive at any given time. States may switch the executive rapidly.

Inner Strength: The one ego state manifestation that apparently all persons have. This ego state claims to have been born with the person, and claims to have wisdom concerning the best direction for the person. It normally speaks with a strong, clear voice, and may call itself by other names, such as "inner self" or "spiritual self".

Internal Communication: Ego states within a single individual communicating with each other. The person may be conscious of this communication; aware of a mental discussion, a decision making weighing of choices, or an argument. The person may also be unconscious of this communication when underlying ego states are communicating. Hypnosis may be required to become aware that this unconscious communication has occurred.

Introject: An introject is an internal manifestation of a person significant in the life of the client. A five-year-old ego state (of an adult client) may have an introject of 'father' or 'mother' as they were at the time the client was five. An introject may also represent another person as they are currently. For example, there may be an introject of a partner, friend, or parent. Introjects may be of living or dead persons, of persons who were viewed as positive or negative, but they are of persons who are or have been meaningful in the life of the client.

Malevolent Ego State: A malevolent ego state is a state that appears to purposely act in opposition to either other (ego) states of the person, or to the outside world. While all ego states start to benefit or protect the individual, over time malevolent states have taken on a negative function. They may learn to assume a positive function, with Ego State Therapy negotiation.

Mapping Ego States: A therapist uses hypnosis to learn the particular ego states of a client. This process includes learning the internal relationships of the states, and the roles of the states. After mapping, a client will be able to have a better self-understanding, and will most often be able to call to the executive the preferred state for a particular situation.

Multiple Personality: *See* Dissociative Identity Disorder

Neurotic Reactions: A situational neurosis is when a client often reacts in an inappropriate manner to a given situation. The neurotic reaction is the inappropriate response that constitutes this pattern. An example of a neurotic reaction is, as part of a pattern, becoming emotionally distressed when criticized by an authority figure. Neurotic reactions are negative feelings of an underlying ego state; feelings from an unresolved issue. When a situational occurrence reminds this ego state of the original unresolved issue, that state temporarily becomes executive with the same feelings of the original occurrence. The client is only aware of experiencing the unwanted reaction.

Obsessive Compulsive Disorder: A psychological disorder characterized by obsessive thought and compulsive action. The client is often unable to control these thoughts and actions, which are often disruptive. For example, an obsessive compulsive client may worry so much about the doors being locked the doors may be checked repeatedly over a relatively short period of time.

Panic Attack: A panic attack is a temporary 'sense of loss of control' and fear, sometimes associated with an inability to have normal function. Panic attacks result from an ego state coming to the executive that has, either unresolved trauma from a past experience, or that has consistently absorbed frustration and anger due to non-assertive expression. Panic attacks may also result from an interactive combination of these two. Each of the two situations result in an ego state feeling overwhelmed and unable to cope, and when this ego state comes to the executive the severe loss of control is experienced.

Protector States: States that were formed to keep the person from experiencing pain. They often help protect fragile states from being hurt, by either keeping them from the executive, or by reacting in a defensive manner, such as with anger or withdrawal. Protector states may also attempt to protect surface states from pain held by underlying states by attempting to keep them buried.

Psychosomatic Symptoms: A physical or medical symptom caused by a psychological phenomenon.

Resistance Bridge Technique: The Resistance Bridge Technique is a hypnotic technique that assists the client in moving directly from the later stages of induction to the origin of the presenting concern. It is used to address unresolved issues. It combines two techniques, the *Resistance*

Deepening Technique, and the *Affect Bridge.* The *Resistance Deepening Technique* uses the client's resistance to hypnosis as a focus to achieve a medium to deep hypnotic state, and the *Affect Bridge* assists clients in moving from the unwanted symptom to the origin of the symptom.

Resistance Deepening Technique: This is a hypnotic deepening technique used in the final stages of induction. It uses the resistance of the client to hypnosis as a focus to deepen the hypnotic state. The *Resistance Deepening Technique* takes what the client cannot keep from focusing upon (resistance), and at the appropriate time, uses that as the primary focus. The hypnotherapist may combine it with most inductions.

Self Talk for Health: An ego state technique where the individual uses self-hypnosis to communicate with an ego state that may have information concerning good health practice. For example, an individual may use *Self Talk for Health* to ask an underlying ego state how to keep the early symptoms of a common cold from continuing to develop into a cold. The internal communication is between an ego state interested in good health, and an ego state with information important to achieving that goal.

Surface States: Surface states are those states that are most often executive in normal daily function. They have good communication between each other. This means that a surface state that is cognitive and deliberative will remember what happened when a surface state that is more emotional was executive. Likewise, a surface emotional state will have good awareness of what happened when the cognitive state was executive. Daily routine is experienced by surface states. Clinically, surface states may be accessed without hypnosis.

Switching: When an ego state is in the executive and a different ego state becomes the executive state switching has occurred.

Underlying States: Underlying states are states that come to the executive rarely. They vary greatly in their relative closeness to the surface. Some very rarely become executive. Some have almost no communication with surface states. These states become executive only occasionally outside of therapy. The person who sees a type of wallpaper like that of a childhood room may experience an underlying ego state, bringing childhood feelings and memories. Some of these memories may have previously been unknown to the surface states. Clinically, underlying states are difficult to access without hypnosis. While most underlying states hold positive and pleasant memories, unresolved trauma is held in underlying states.